CW00382837

Vegetarian

Table of Contents

Book 1

Introduction..2
Vegetable Quesadillas on Whole-Wheat Tortillas 3
Roasted Beets with Grapefruit Glaze 4
Chard with Onion and Tamari 5
Roasted Curried Cauliflower Recipe 6
Mushroom & Tomato Appetizers 7
Pan Roasted Baby Artichokes with Pistachios, Lemon and Black Quinoa.............8
Cuban Black Bean Stew with Rice 9
Vegetarian Dan-Dan Noodles 10
Veggie Red Thai Curry 11
Sweet and Sour Cabbage Wedges...12
Roasted Delicata Squash with Kale 13
Steamed Artichoke..14
Spicy Vegetarian Tortilla Soup Recipe...15
Butternut Squash Casserole 16
Veggie Udon Noodle Soup 17
Cream of Cauliflower Soup 18
Black Bean, Corn and Tomatillo Salad...19
Sesame Tofu 20
Seitan Stew 21
Potato Salad 22
Spicy Jalapeno Black Bean Burgers 23
Stir-Fried Tofu with Scallions...24
Brown Rice Salad 25
Falafel with Avocado Spread..26
Tomato, Zucchini, White Bean, and Basil Soup 27
Vegetable Jalfrezi 28
Braised Radishes...30
Quick and Easy Springtime Sorrel Soup...31
Secret Smokey Split Peas..32
Spaghetti and Vegetarian Meatballs 33
Vegetarian Korean Pancakes 35
Spent Grain Burgers..36
Zesty Wheat Berry Black Bean Chili..37
Chinese-Style Eggplant...38
Cumin-Spiced Chickpeas and Carrots on Couscous 39
Blackened Tofu Po'Boys 40
Stuffed Grape Leaves..41

Book 2

Introduction 43

Chapter 1 Vegan Breakfasts Galore 44

Chapter 2 Lunch Break Time 54

Chapter 3 Dinner Must Haves 21. Roasted 68

10-Week Vegetarian Smart Cookbook Book 1

Introduction

This book contains proven steps and strategies on how to eat a vegetarian diet for the next ten weeks.

Consuming a vegetarian diet has shown potential for improving focus, energy, and overall health in individuals who do not obtain enough nutrition from their current diets. Those who eat out often and lack a regular consumption of vegetables and fruits in their everyday diet will benefit from consuming a vegetarian diet. Not only will vegetarianism help you boost your overall intake of vitamins and minerals, but it can also help protect you from major diseases!

There is evidence that vegetarians are at a lower risk of cardiac events like heart attacks and heart arrhythmias. In one study that involved more than seventy-six thousand participants, vegetarians were twenty-five percent less likely to die from heart disease. In addition, vegetarians are also less likely to develop certain types of cancer. Hundreds of studies have suggested consuming more fruits and vegetables will reduce the risk of cancer developing in the body. Lastly, eating more fruits and vegetables puts you at a lower risk of type 2 diabetes. Research has shown that a mostly plant-based diet is able to reduce the risk for type to diabetes because consuming more plants means more fiber, and more fiber means a healthier colon and healthier weight.

Therefore, eating a vegetarian diet is much healthier for you than eating red meat and potatoes for dinner. So let's dive into some just as filling, but much healthier, alternatives to the norm!

Vegetable Quesadillas on Whole-Wheat Tortillas

Serves: 4-5

Ingredients

- 2 Tbsp. Olive Oil
- ½ C. Onion, Diced
- 2 C. Mixed Veggies, Diced
- ¾ Tsp. Chili Powder
- 1 Lime, Juiced
- Salt
- 2 C. Cheese, Grated
- 6 Whole-Wheat Tortillas
- Butter
- Avocado
- Sour Cream
- Cilantro
- Salsa
- Hot Peppers

Directions

1. Heat the oil in a pan over medium heat and toss in the onion and diced vegetables. Cook for four to five minutes or until they're tender.
2. Add the Chile, lime, and salt to the vegetable mix.
3. Heat a griddle to 375 degrees.
4. In a bowl, mix the vegetables with the cheese and spread a thin layer on three tortillas. Top them with the remaining tortillas.
5. Melt the butter on your griddle and cook the quesadillas for a few minutes or until they start to brown.
6. Repeat on the other side until it's lightly browned.
7. Let it cool a few minutes before you cut it.
8. Serve with the toppings and enjoy.

Roasted Beets with Grapefruit Glaze

Serves: 4-6

Ingredients

- 3 Lbs. Beets
- 1 C. -Squeezed Grapefruit Juice
- 1 Tbsp. Rice Vinegar
- 3 Scant Tbsp. Pure Maple Syrup
- 1 Tbsp. Corn Starch

Directions

1. Preheat your oven to 450 degrees Fahrenheit.
2. Trim the stems off the beets and divide them into two groups. Put them on two large pieces of foil and drizzle with two tablespoons of water. Fold into a packet and put it on the center oven rack for an hour. Check after forty minutes if you have small beets.
3. When they can be pierced with a fork, they're done. Remove them from the oven and the foil packets. Allow them to cool until you can handle them without burning yourself. Trim off the rest of the stem and rub them to gently peel off the skin.
4. Slice the beets thinly.
5. Whisk the juice through the syrup together in a bowl.
6. Measure the starch into a pan and whisk the liquids into it slowly to avoid any clumps.
7. Once the juice is added and it's starting to get thick, reduce the heat and stir it often for five minutes.
8. Serve the glaze over the hot beets and serve immediately.

Chard with Onion and Tamari

Serves: 2-3

Ingredients

- 1 Bunch Chard, Coarsely Chopped
- 1 Small Onion, Chopped
- Tamari

Directions

1. In a skillet, sauté the onion until it's tender, around five minutes.
2. Add the chard and sauté that until it's a bright green and becomes a little limp.
3. Season with the tamari and heat it through.
4. Serve.

Roasted Curried Cauliflower Recipe

Serves: 2-4

Ingredients

- 2 Lbs. Cauliflower
- Curry Powder
- Olive Oil
- Sea Salt

Directions

1. Preheat your oven to 500 degrees Fahrenheit. Break the cauliflower into small florets and put it in a bowl. Be sure the pieces are as even as possible.
2. Drizzle them with the oil and season with the curry powder and salt. Place them in a single layer on the bottom of a baking pan.
3. Cover with foil and put it in the oven. Roast for ten to fifteen minutes covered, and then remove the foil and toss them with some tongs. Continue to stir them every eight to ten minutes or until the tips start to become crispy. This should take around half an hour.
4. Adjust the seasonings and serve.

Mushroom & Tomato Appetizers

Serves: 8

Ingredients

- 10 Oz. Frozen Spinach
- 1 Lb. Cremini Mushrooms
- 1 Lb. Cherry Tomatoes
- 6 Oz. Feta Cheese
- 5 Garlic Cloves, Minced
- ¼ C. Green Onion, Minced
- 4 Tbsp. Extra Virgin Olive Oil
- 2-3 Tbsp. Basil, Chopped
- Salt
- Pepper
- Parmesan Cheese

Directions

1. Defrost the spinach and drain it thoroughly. Press it with the paper towels to get out as much moisture as possible.
2. Open up the cherry tomatoes about a third of the way down and clean out the insides with a melon baller.
3. Wash the mushrooms and remove the stems. Mince up a quarter cup of the stems.
4. Sauté the garlic, stems, and onion in the oil and add the spinach. Add the basil and season to taste. Cool before you add the feta.
5. To assemble, put a tablespoon of the filling into the mushroom caps and tomatoes.
6. Arrange on an oiled baking sheet and put it in a 350 degree Fahrenheit oven for twenty minutes. Top with the cheese and serve over some lettuce.

Pan Roasted Baby Artichokes with Pistachios, Lemon and Black Quinoa
Serves: 2

Ingredients

- 1 Lb. Small Artichokes
- ½ Shallot
- ¼ C. Pistachio Nuts, Shelled
- 1 Lemon, Juiced And Zested
- ½ C. Black Quinoa, Cooked
- ¼ C. + 1 Tbsp. Olive Oil
- Salt And Pepper

Directions

1. Start the quinoa first.
2. Whisk a quarter cup of the oil, lemon juice, and a bit of salt in a mixing bowl. Clean the artichokes and remove the tough leaves.
3. Cut the artichoke in half and submerge it in the lemon and olive mix. As you clean the artichokes and add them to the mix, be sure to stir the bowl every now and gain to make sure they don't remain exposed to the air too long. They will turn black through the process of oxidation if you forget to do this.
4. Slice the shallot thinly and heat a tablespoon of the oil in a pan over medium heat. Once it swirls in the pan easily, add the nuts and shallot. Once the shallot starts to brown, toss in the zest and stir. Cook for another minute.
5. Add the artichokes and their liquid to the pan and season them to taste. Turn them so the faces are touching the surface of the pan and let them brown on one side as the liquid reduces. Stir them every few minutes to let the liquid almost reduce completely. If the pan dries out before your artichokes are cooked, then add a third of a cup of water to prevent them from burning.
6. Once the artichokes are done, meaning they're tender all the way through, toss in the quinoa and mix it well. Be sure to scrape the bits of shallot and the zest into the quinoa. Season to taste and serve.

Cuban Black Bean Stew with Rice

Serves: 4

Ingredients

- 1 C. Uncooked Brown Rice
- 1 Tbsp. Olive Oil
- 1 Red Onion, Diced
- 1 Red Bell Pepper, Diced
- 1 Green Pepper, Diced
- 2 Garlic Cloves, Minced
- 3 C. Black Beans, Rinsed And Drained
- 1 ½ C. Vegetable Broth
- 1 Tbsp. Apple Cider Vinegar
- 1 Bay Leaf
- 1 Tsp. Dried Oregano
- ½ Tsp. Ground Cumin
- ½ C. Frozen Corn Kernels
- ¼ Bunch Cilantro
- Salt And Pepper

Directions

1. Combine the rice with two cups of water in a pot and bring it to a boil. Reduce the heat and allow it to simmer for forty minutes. Let it stand for five minutes.
2. Heat the oil in a pan and sauté the peppers through the garlic for ten minutes.
3. Add the beans through the cumin and mince the cilantro. Add the cilantro and season with salt and pepper.
4. Allow it to simmer and then mash the beans with the back of a spoon. Stir in the corn and return it to a simmer.
5. Adjust the seasonings as needed and serve over the rice. Garnish with a bit more cilantro.

Vegetarian Dan-Dan Noodles

Serves: 4-6

Ingredients

- 2 Dried Shiitake Mushrooms
- 4 Oz. Crumbled, Thawed Extra-Firm Tofu
- 1 Tsp. Peppercorns
- 2 Tsp. Plus 1 Tbsp. Soy Sauce
- ½ Tsp. Plus 1 Tbsp. Dark Soy Sauce
- 2 Tbsp. Sesame Paste
- 2 Tbsp. Chile Oil
- Salt
- 1 ½ Tbsp. Canola Oil
- 4 Dried Chiles
- 2 Tbsp. Minced Dill Pickle
- 1 Lb. Chinese Noodles
- 1 Scallion, Green Part Sliced

Directions

1. Soak the mushroom in some water to rehydrate it. Stem and mince the mushrooms. Put them into a small bowl and add the tofu. Season with two teaspoons of the soy sauce and half a teaspoon of the dark soy sauce. Set them aside.
2. In a skillet, toast the peppercorns until they're fragrant and starting to smoke a bit. Set them aside to cool before pounding them into a coarse texture with a spice grinder or mortar and pestle.
3. To make the sauce, combine half the peppercorns with a tablespoon of soy sauce in a bowl. Then add a tablespoon of dark soy sauce, the paste, and the Chile oil. Divide this among bowls or put it in one big bowl and set it aside.
4. To make the tofu topping, heat the oil in a wok over medium heat and add the Chile with the remaining peppercorns and stir-fry until they're fragrant, around fifteen seconds. Add the mushroom and tofu mix and preserve the pickle. Cook until it's warmed through, around two minutes. Remove it from the heat and set it aside.
5. Cook the noodles in unsalted water and drain them with water to remove any excess starch. Add the noodles to the bowls and stir them to coat. Top with the stir-fried mix, scallion, and serve.

Veggie Red Thai Curry
Serves: 3-4

Ingredients

- 1 Tbsp. Coconut Oil
- 2 Garlic Cloves, Minced
- ½ Sweet Onion, Sliced
- 4 Tbsp. Thai Red Curry Paste
- 1 Can Coconut Milk
- ½ C. Water
- 2 Tbsp. Tamari
- 1 ½ Tbsp. Coconut Palm Sugar
- 1 Zucchini, Chopped
- 1 Sweet Potato, Cubed
- 8 Mushrooms, Sliced
- 1" Piece Of Ginger, Sliced
- ½ Red Pepper, Sliced
- 1 Bunch Of Thai Basil, Shredded
- 1 Lime, Cut Into Wedges

Directions

1. In a pan, add the oil and sauté the garlic and onions for five minutes.
2. Add the curry paste and stir it in. pour in the milk through the sugar and stir it to combine. Then bring it to a boil.
3. Toss in the vegetables and ginger and reduce the heat to simmer for fifteen to twenty minutes.
4. Serve over rice or quinoa with the basil and lime as a garnish.

Sweet and Sour Cabbage Wedges

Serves: 4

Ingredients

- 2 Tbsp. Olive Oil
- ½ Head Green Cabbage, Quartered
- ½ C. Cider Vinegar
- 2 Tbsp. Sugar
- Salt And Pepper

Directions

1. In a skillet, heat the oil. Add the cabbage and cook for two to four minutes on either side.
2. Add the vinegar and sugar with one and a half cups of water. Bring it to a simmer and cook until the cabbage has become tender, around twelve to fifteen minutes.
3. Season to taste and serve.

Roasted Delicata Squash with Kale

Serves: 2

Ingredients

- 1 Medium Delicata Squash
- 1 Bunch Kale
- 1 Garlic Clove
- 2 Tbsp. Olive Oil, Divided
- Salt And Pepper

Directions

1. Preheat your oven to 425 degrees Fahrenheit and scrub the squash to clean it. Slice the ends off and it in half the long direction. Scoop out the seeds with a melon baller and cut it into half-moon shapes or quarters that are no more than half an inch thick.
2. Toss it with a tablespoon of oil and arrange it on a baking sheet in a single layer. Roast it for twenty minutes, turning halfway through.
3. As the squash roasts, remove the stems from the kale and rinse it. Chop it and then chop a garlic clove.
4. Heat the other half of the oil in a pan and sauté the kale with a pinch of salt. Add the garlic and cook another minute. Then add two tablespoons of water and stir it briefly before removing it from the heat.
5. Serve the squash over the greens and season with salt and pepper to taste.

Steamed Artichoke

Serves: 1

Ingredients

- 1 Large Artichoke
- ¼ Lemon
- Olive Oil
- Salt
- Chopped Parsley
- Lemon Oil

Directions

1. With a sharp knife, cut off the top of the artichoke. Peel off the bottom leaves and use scissors to trim off the thorn tips of the rest of the leaves. Use the knife to cut the stem off the bulb and make sure the artichoke sits up straight.
2. Fill a stock pot with half an inch of water and bring it to a boil. Put the artichoke with the face down into the water, reduce your heat to a simmer, and cover it with a lid. Steam for twenty minutes without lifting the lid.
3. Once it's finished, use tongs to turn the artichoke so it's sitting upright. Drizzle oil over it and then sprinkle with salt. Add another cup of water and cover it again. Steam another twenty minutes.
4. Use the tongs to remove the artichoke to a serving platter.
5. Squeeze the lemon over the leaves and sprinkle it with parsley. Serve.

Spicy Vegetarian Tortilla Soup Recipe

Serves: 2-3

Ingredients

- 2 Tbsp. Olive Oil
- 1 Onion, Chopped
- 6 Garlic Cloves, Minced
- 3 Jalapeno Peppers, Seeded And Chopped
- 1 Tbsp. Cumin Seed
- 1 C. Corn Kernels
- 2 29 Oz. Cans Vegetable Broth
- 2 16 Oz. Cans Kidney Beans, Rinsed And Drained
- ⅓ C. Cilantro, Chopped
- 1 C. Monterey Jack Cheese, Shredded
- 6 Corn Tortillas
- Cooking Spray
- Sour Cream
- Lime Wedges

Directions

1. Add the oil through the cumin seed to a pot over medium heat and sauté for five minutes. Add the corn through the cilantro and reduce the heat to a simmer for ten minutes.
2. Heat your oven to 450 degrees Fahrenheit and coat a cookie sheet with some cooking spray. Put the tortillas on the sheet and spray them with the cooking spray. Cook for ten minutes. Cut them into strips.
3. Top the soup with the cheese, strips, and a dollop of sour cream. Garnish with a lime wedge.

Butternut Squash Casserole

Serves: 2-4

Ingredients

- 1 Butternut Squash
- 3 Tbsp. Maple Syrup
- 15 Oz. Black Beans
- ½ Leek, Chopped
- ½ Sweet Onion, Chopped
- Himalayan Salt
- ⅓ Loaf Sourdough Bread
- 2 Tbsp. Butter

Directions

1. Cut the squash into quarters and remove the seeds. Wrap them in foil packets and bake for forty minutes or until they're just soft. Remove the meat from them with a spoon. Mash it with the maple syrup and a little salt.
2. Sauté the onions and leek in a pan for three minutes.
3. Cut the bread into small pieces and toss it with the melted butter.
4. Layer the squash with the beans, leeks, and onions in a two-quart glass baking dish.
5. Put the croutons on the top.
6. Bake for twenty minutes uncovered at 350 degrees Fahrenheit. Serve hot and enjoy.

Veggie Udon Noodle Soup
Serves: 4-6

Ingredients

- 3 C. Vegetable Broth
- 1 Zucchini, Chopped
- 1 C. Broccoli, Chopped
- 6 Mushrooms, Sliced
- 1 Carrot, Chopped
- 2 Garlic Cloves, Minced
- 3 Tbsp. Tamari
- 1 Package Udon Noodles
- Cayenne Pepper
- Red Pepper Flakes
- Salt

Directions

1. Cook the noodles according to their package directions. Drain and rinse them with cold water, then set them aside. Add a bit of vegetable broth so they don't stick.
2. In another pot, add the broth through the garlic. Bring it to a low boil and the simmer for five to ten minutes. Add the udon noodles, along with seasonings to your taste and stir.
3. Pour the soup into bowls and season with a little extra red pepper flakes.

Cream of Cauliflower Soup

Serves: 2

Ingredients

- ½ Onion
- ½ Garlic Clove
- 1 Potato
- ½ Cauliflower Head
- ½ Carrot
- ¼ C. Oats Milk
- 2" Stalk Of Celery, Chopped
- Pinch Of Dill
- Half A Bay Leaf

Directions

1. Sauté the onion and garlic in a pot until it's translucent. Add the potato and carrot and cook a little more.
2. Add the water, cauliflower, celery, a little dill, and a half a bay leaf. Allow this to boil for fifteen minutes. Blend and then add the milk. Warm it again after you've added the milk and enjoy.

Black Bean, Corn and Tomatillo Salad

Serves: 2

Ingredients

- 1 Can Black Beans, Rinsed And Drained
- 1 ½ C. Corn Kernels
- 1 C. Chopped Tomatillos
- ¼ C. Raw Pumpkin Seeds
- ¾ C. Chives
- 1 Avocado, Chopped
- 3 Tbsp. Lemon Juice
- 2 Tbsp. Olive Oil
- ½ Tsp. Ground Cumin
- Salt
- Pepper

Directions

1. Mix the beans through the avocado together in a bowl.
2. Mix together the lemon juice through the pepper together in a separate bowl and whisk together.
3. Add the first bowl to the second bowl and mix well. Enjoy.

Sesame Tofu

Serves: 3-4

Ingredients

- 1 Package Extra Firm Tofu, Cubed
- 2 Tbsp. Cornstarch
- 1 Tsp. Garlic Powder
- ½ Tsp. Ground Ginger
- ¼ Tsp. Cayenne Pepper
- Canola Oil
- 4 Tbsp. Soy Sauce
- 2 Tbsp. Honey
- 1 Tbsp. Minced Garlic
- 1 Tbsp. Sesame Oil
- 1 Tsp. Gochu Garu
- 2 Scallion Stems, Chopped
- 2 Tbsp. Sesame Seeds

Directions

1. In a container, add the cornstarch through the cayenne. Once they're combined, add the tofu and seal it with a lid or some plastic wrap. Shake it until the cubes are evenly coated with the mix.
2. Add the oil to the frying pan and heat it. Brown the tofu cubes on all sides. Move them onto a paper towel so it can absorb any extra oil.
3. In the pan you used to fry the cubes, add the sauce through the pepper flakes. Once it's warmed, stir together and add the tofu cubes back in. Stir them around in the glaze.
4. Once they're glazed, add the seeds and serve with the chopped scallions over some rice or vegetables.

Seitan Stew
Serves: 1-2

Ingredients

- 1 Carrot
- ½ Onion
- ¼ C. Peas
- ½ Eggplant
- 4 White Button Mushrooms
- ½ Tomato
- Seitan
- ½ Bay Leaf
- Salt
- Olive Oil

Directions

1. Chop the onion and carrot and sauté them until they're tender. Add the peas and the eggplant and sauté another five minutes.
2. Add some water along with the seiten through the tomato and bring it to a boil.
3. Reduce the heat to a simmer and cook twenty minutes.
4. Serve.

Potato Salad

Serves: 5

Ingredients

- 5 C. Of Potatoes, Chopped And Boiled
- 2 Ears Of Corn, Kernels Removed And Cooked
- 1 Red Pepper, Grilled
- 1 Zucchini, Grilled
- ½ Head Of Radicchio
- 1 C. Chives, Chopped
- ⅓ C. Pine Nuts, Toasted
- 1 C. Basil, Chopped
- 1 C. Feta Cheese, Crumbled
- ½ C. Olive Oil
- ⅓ C. Balsamic Vinegar
- 1 Tbsp. Sucanat
- Pepper

Directions

1. Whisk the olive oil through the pepper to taste together. Once the ingredients are prepared to their directions, toss them with the dressing a bit at a time.
2. Serve.

Spicy Jalapeno Black Bean Burgers

Serves: 6

Ingredients

- 15 Oz. Cooked Black Beans
- ½ C. Pecans, Diced
- ½ Medium Onion, Diced Finely
- 4 Cloves Garlic, Minced
- 1 Jalapeno Pepper, Minced
- 1 Tsp. Ground Cumin
- ½ Tbsp. Miso Paste
- 1 Tbsp. Adobo Sauce
- 1 Tbsp. Tomato Paste
- 1 Tsp. Kosher Salt
- ½ Tsp. Black Pepper
- ½ Tbsp. Dried Parsley
- 1 Tsp. Dried Oregano
- 1 Tbsp. Flax Seeds
- 1 Tbsp. Wheat Germ
- 1 Egg White
- ⅓ C. Whole Wheat Flour
- Oil For Frying

Directions

1. Put the bean in a bowl and mash them with the back of a spoon or a potato masher. You want them broken but not mashed up completely.
2. Add the nuts through the egg white and mix it well with a spoon or your hands. Add the flour in last and fold it in until it's combined. Chill this mix for ten minutes.
3. Put a skillet over high heat and when the pan's hot, add a tablespoon of oil.
4. Use a third of a cup-measuring cup and scoop the bean mix into balls. Then flatten and put into the pan. Cook for three to five minutes on either side until it's crisp.
5. Serve on a bun with your favorite toppings.

Stir-Fried Tofu with Scallions

Serves: 4

Ingredients

- 1 ½ To 2 Lbs. Firm To Extra-Firm Tofu, Dried
- 3 Tbsp. Peanut Oil
- 1 Tbsp. Garlic, Chopped
- 1 Tbsp. Ginger, Chopped And Peeled
- 2 Dried Chiles
- 2 C. Chopped Scallions, Green And White Parts
- ⅓ C. Vegetable Stock
- 2 Tbsp. Soy Sauce
- 1 Tbsp. Toasted Sesame Seeds

Directions

1. Cut the tofu into half inch cubes and put the oil in a skillet over high heat. Add the garlic, ginger, and chili and sauté for ten seconds. Add the tofu and the whites of the scallions, sautéing them until the tofu starts to brown. Add the stock and stir it as it cooks until about half has evaporated. Add the green parts of the scallions and stir for thirty seconds.
2. Add the soy and adjust the seasonings to taste. Serve.

Brown Rice Salad

Serves: 2

Ingredients

- 2 C. Cooked Brown Rice
- ⅓ C. Cooked Black Beans, Drained And Rinsed
- ¼ C. Raisins
- 4 Scallions
- 2 Tsp. Champagne Or Wine Vinegar
- ¼ Tsp. Kosher Salt
- ¼ Tsp. Dijon Mustard
- 3 Tbsp. Olive Oil
- ¼ C. Chopped Almonds
- Black Pepper

Directions

1. Stir the rice and beans together. Slice the scallions and separate the light and dark pieces.
2. Combine the light parts of the scallions with the raisins through the salt. Whisk the oil in until it's emulsified.
3. Pour the dressing over the beans and rice and mix it thoroughly. Add a bit more oil if it seems to dry.
4. Cover and allow it to stand for half an hour.
5. Top with some almonds and pepper. Serve cold.

Falafel with Avocado Spread

Serves: 4

Ingredients

- 15 Oz. Can Pinto Beans
- ½ C Monterey Jack Cheese, Shredded
- ¼ C. Tortilla Chips, Crushed
- 2 Tbsp. Green Onions, Minced
- 1 Tbsp. Cilantro, Minced
- ⅛ Tsp. Ground Cumin
- Egg White
- 1 ½ Tsp. Canola Oil
- ¼ C. Avocado, Mashed And Peeled
- Tbsp. Tomato, Minced
- 1 Tbsp. Red Onion, Minced
- Tbsp. Sour Cream
- 1 Tsp. Lime Juice
- ⅛ Tsp. Salt
- 2 Pitas, Halved
- Red Onion Slices, Separated Into Rings
- Microgreens

Directions

1. To make the patties, place the beans in a bowl and mash them with a fork. Add the cheese and the following five ingredients. Stir until it's well combined. Shape into four half inch oval patties.
2. Heat the oil in a skillet over medium heat and cook the patties for three minutes on either side.
3. To make the spread, combine the avocado with the following five ingredients and stir well. Put one patty in a patty half and spread two tablespoons of the avocado mix over the patties in the pitas. Top with the greens and onion slices.

Tomato, Zucchini, White Bean, and Basil Soup

Serves: 1

Ingredients

- ¼ C. White Beans
- Olive Oil
- ¼ C. Zucchini, Chopped
- ¼ Tomato, Chopped
- Dried Thyme
- Basil Leaves

Directions

1. Soak the beans in water overnight.
2. Sauté the onion and garlic and boil the soaked beans in water seasoned with thyme for one hour.
3. Add the chopped zucchini and the tomatoes and boil for ten more minutes. Season with the basil leaves.
4. Serve.

Vegetable Jalfrezi

Serves: 1

Ingredients

- 1 Onion
- 1 Fred Chilli
- 1" Piece Ginger
- 2 Garlic Cloves
- 1 Small Bunch Coriander
- 1 Cauliflower
- 2 Red Peppers
- 1 Small Butternut Squash
- 3 Ripe Tomatoes
- 14 Oz. Canned Chickpeas
- Vegetable Oil
- 1 Tbsp. Butter
- 8 Oz. Curry Paste
- 28 Oz. Canned Chopped Tomatoes
- 4 Tbsp. Balsamic Vinegar
- Sea Salt
- Pepper
- 2 Lemons
- 7 Oz. Plain Yoghurt

Directions

1. To make the curry, peel and halve the onion. Chop the onion and slice the chili finely. Peel and slice the ginger and garlic finely. Pick the coriander leaves and chop the stalks. Halve and chop the peppers.
2. Break the cauliflower into florets and chop them. Quarter the tomatoes.
3. Halve the squash and scoop out the seeds. Slice the squash into wedges and leave the peel on, but remove any thick areas of the skin. Roughly chop it into smaller pieces and drain the chickpeas.
4. Put a casserole pan on medium high heat and add a few tablespoons of oil as well as the butter. Add the chopped onion, chili, ginger, garlic, and the cilantro stalks. Sauté for ten minutes until it's softened and browned. Add the peppers along with the squash, chickpeas, and curry past. Stir well to coat all the vegetables with the paste.

5. Add the cauliflower and the tomatoes to the dish. Then add the vinegar and add fourteen ounces of water to the pan.
6. Bring it to a boil and turn the heat down to a simmer for forty-five minutes, covered. Check after half an hour. If it still looks too runny, leave the lid off for the last fifteen minutes.
7. When the vegetables are tender, season to taste and squeeze the lemon juice over it.
8. Garnish with a dollop of yogurt and a sprinkle of cilantro leaves.

Braised Radishes

Serves: 4

Ingredients

- 20 Radishes
- 2 Tbsp. Butter, Divided
- 1 Shallot, Diced
- 1 Tsp. Chopped Thyme
- Salt And Pepper
- 3 Tbsp. White Wine

Directions

1. Remove the leaves from the radishes and leave a bit of the green stems. Reserve the leaves if they're in good condition and scrub the radishes. Leave the small ones whole and cut any large ones in half.
2. In a sauté pan, melt the butter over medium heat and sauté the shallots and thyme for a minute. Add the radishes, a bit of salt, and enough water to cover them.
3. Simmer until the radishes are tender, around three to five minutes. Add the leaves and cook for one minute or until they've wilted. Remove them to a serving dish.
4. Bring the liquid to a boil and add the wine. Reduce it to about a quarter of a cup and pour this over the radishes. Season with pepper and serve.

Quick and Easy Springtime Sorrel Soup

Serves: 2

Ingredients

- 1 Tbsp. Olive Oil
- ½ Onion, Chopped
- 2 Packed C. Chopped Sorrel, Stems Removed
- 2 C. Vegetable Broth
- ¼ Tsp. Salt
- ½ C. Plain Yogurt
- 2 Tbsp. Chopped Cashews
- 2 Tbsp. Chopped Cilantro

Directions

1. Heat the oil in a two-quart pot over medium heat and sauté the onions until they're translucent. Add the sorrel and sauté until it's wilted. Add the stock and bring it to a boil. Simmer for seven to ten minutes and remove it from the heat.
2. Use an immersion blender to puree the soup. Season with salt, if needed.
3. Swirl in the yogurt and ladle it into bowls. Top with some chopped cashews and chopped cilantro. Serve.

Secret Smokey Split Peas

Serves: 6-8

Ingredients

- 1 Onion, Chopped
- ½ Garlic Clove, Diced
- 1 Turnip, Peeled And Chopped
- 3 Chopped Carrots
- 2 Tbsp. Olive Oil
- 1 Tbsp. Thyme
- 1 ¼ C. Soy Sauce
- 2 Tbsp. Vegetable Bullion Paste
- 3 C. Split Peas
- 6 C. Water
- Chipotle Peppers In Adobo Sauce, To Taste

Directions

1. Sauté the vegetable in the oil over medium heat for twenty minutes. Add the thyme toward the end.
2. Chop half the peppers and add them to the pan along with three tablespoons of the sauce. Sauté for five more minutes. Turn the heat up high and deglaze the pan with the soy sauce.
3. Add the peas, water, and bullion
4. After it comes to a boil, turn the heat down to a simmer and stir every now and again. Simmer for an hour and serve.

Spaghetti and Vegetarian Meatballs

Serves: 4-6

Ingredients

- ¼ C. Olive Oil
- 1 C. Onion, Chopped
- 3 Cloves Garlic, Chopped
- ¼ Tsp Crushed Red Pepper
- ½ C. Red Wine
- 6 Oz. Can Tomato Paste
- 28 Oz. Can Crushed Tomatoes
- 4 C. Water
- 1 C. Green Pepper, Chopped
- 2 Bay Leaves
- 1 Tbsp. Oregano
- 2 Tsp. Basil
- 1 Tsp. Marjoram
- 1 Tsp. Fennel Seed
- 1 Tsp. Sugar
- 1 ¼ Tsp. Sea Salt
- Pepper
- 2" Parmesan Rind
- 1 Lb. Spaghetti
- Grated Parmesan, For Serving
- 14 Oz. Sausage Flavored Tofu
- ½ C. Dry Bread Crumbs
- ½ C. Parmesan, Grated
- 1 Egg
- ½ Cup Parsley, Chopped
- 2 Tbsp. Olive Oil

Directions

1. Add the fourteen ounces of sausage tofu through the parsley into a food processor.
2. Process everything until it's incorporated and stop to scrape down the bowl a few times.
3. Heat the oil in a saucepan and make balls with your hands.
4. Scrape out the desired amount and roll it into a ball. Then set it aside on a plate.
5. Place them in the heated oil and cook them until they're lightly browned, turning a few times, about eight to ten minutes.

6. Remove them to a plate to drain.
7. Then heat up some more oil in the pan and sauté the onion until it's lightly browned about ten minutes. Add the garlic and the crushed red pepper and cook it another minute.
8. Add the wine and stir it to scrape up any browned bits. Bring it to a simmer.
9. Stir in the paste and cook for another minute.
10. Stir in the tomatoes, water, pepper, bay, basil, oregano, fennel, marjoram, salt, sugar, and pepper. Add the parmesan rind and bring it to a boil. Reduce the heat to a simmer for an hour and cover partially. Add more water if it becomes too thick.
11. Stir the meatballs into the sauce and bring it to a boil. Reduce the heat and simmer it again for ten more minutes. Remove the parmesan rind and the bay leaves.
12. Bring a pot of water to a boil and cook the pasta according to its directions. Drain and serve with the sauce and meatballs.

Vegetarian Korean Pancakes

Serves: 2

Ingredients

- 1 C. All-Purpose Flour
- 1 C. Rice Flour
- 2 Eggs, Beaten
- 1 ½ C. Cold Water
- 1 Tbsp. Canola Oil
- 1 C. Garlic Chives, Sliced
- ½ C. Carrots, Peeled Cut Into Thin Matchsticks
- ½ C. Shitake Mushrooms, Sliced
- 1 Tbsp. Prepared Kimchi, Chopped
- ¼ C. Soy Sauce
- 3 Tbsp. Rice Vinegar
- ¼ Tsp. Sesame Oil
- 1 Tsp. Sugar
- 2 Tsp. Minced Ginger
- 1 Tsp. Toasted Sesame Seeds

Directions

1. To make the dipping sauce, stir the soy sauce through the sugar in a bowl until the sugar has dissolved. Add the ginger and stir it, crushing the ginger against the side of the bowl as you go. Let it sit for a few minutes and stir in the sesame seeds when you're ready to serve it.
2. In a bowl, combine the flours, egg, water and oil until it's smooth. Let it rest a few moments as you prepare the vegetables.
3. Stir the vegetables and kimchi together and toss them to coat. Heat a skillet over medium heat and coat it with some oil. Once the pan is hot, drop the batter in and make five pancakes. Spread out the batter so it's not more than half an inch thick. Turn the heat down to low. Cook for four minutes, flipping and cooking another four minutes to brown both sides. The pancake should be crispy and brown without any liquid inside.
4. Serve hot with the dipping sauce, some extra kimchi, and hot sauce.

Spent Grain Burgers

Serves: 8

Ingredients

- 1 C. Spent Grain
- 1 C. Cooked Quinoa
- 2 Eggs
- 5 Tbsp. Barbecue Sauce
- ¾ Tsp Salt
- ½ C. Bread Crumbs

Directions

1. Combine everything in a bowl until it's fully mixed. Heat some oil on a griddle.
2. Scoop a handful of the mix into your hands and flatten them to make a patty. Put the patty on the griddle and cook on either side for five to eight minutes.
3. Serve hot.

Zesty Wheat Berry Black Bean Chili

Serves: 4-6

Ingredients

- 2 Tbsp. Extra-Virgin Olive Oil
- 1 Yellow Onion, Chopped
- 1 Yellow Bell Pepper, Chopped
- 5 Garlic Cloves, Minced
- 2 Tsp. Chili Powder
- 1 ½ Tsp. Ground Cumin
- 1 Tsp. Dried Oregano
- ½ Tsp. Salt
- ½ Tsp. Pepper
- 2 15 Oz. Cans Black Beans, Rinsed
- 2 14 Oz. Diced Tomatoes, Undrained
- 2 Canned Chipotle Peppers In Adobo Sauce, Minced
- 2 C. Vegetable Broth
- 2 Tsp. Light Brown Sugar
- 2 C. Cooked Wheat Berries
- Juice Of 1 Lime
- 1 Avocado, Diced
- ½ C. Chopped Cilantro

Directions

1. Heat the oil in a Dutch oven and sauté the onion through the pepper. Cook and stir occasionally for five minutes.
2. Add the beans through the brown sugar and bring it to a boil. Reduce the heat and simmer it for twenty-five minutes.
3. Stir in the wheat berries and heat them through, about five more minutes. Remove it from the heat, stir in the lime juice, and garnish with the avocado and cilantro.

Chinese-Style Eggplant

Serves: 2-3

Ingredients

- 4 Japanese Eggplant
- ½ Tbsp. Coconut Or Peanut Oil
- 1 Garlic Cloves, Minced
- 1 Tbsp. Soy Sauce
- 1 Tsp. Rice Vinegar
- 1 Tsp. Toasted Sesame Oil
- Pinch Red Pepper Flakes
- Sesame Seeds
- Scallions, Chopped

Directions

1. Slice the eggplant in half the long direction. Heat a wok over medium heat and add the oil.
2. Once the oil is almost smoking, add the eggplant in. Flip it once until it's browned, about two minutes on either side.
3. Combine the remainder of the ingredients and two tablespoons of water. Add that to the pan and stir it briefly before covering it to let it steam.
4. Stir it again and add some more water if you need to deglaze the pan.
5. Let it rest five minutes before serving. Garnish with the sesame seeds and the scallions.

Cumin-Spiced Chickpeas and Carrots on Couscous

Serves: 4

Ingredients

- ½ C. Vegetable Broth
- 1 Tbsp. Lemon Rind, Grated
- 3 Tbsp. Lemon Juice
- 1 Tbsp. Tomato Paste
- 2 15 ½ Oz. Cans Chickpeas
- 3 Tbsp. Canola Oil, Divided
- 1 C. Red Bell Pepper, Chopped
- 1 C. Carrots, Sliced
- 1 Jalapeño Pepper, Minced
- 1 Tsp. Cumin Seeds
- ¼ Tsp. Salt
- ¼ Tsp. Black Pepper
- ¼ Tsp. Ground Allspice
- ⅛ Tsp. Ground Red Pepper
- 6 Garlic Cloves, Minced
- 4 C. Cooked Couscous
- ½ C. Cilantro Leaves
- Lemon Wedges

Directions

1. Combine the first four ingredients in a bowl and whisk together.
2. Dry the chickpeas between paper towels and heat two tablespoons of oil in a skillet. Add the chickpeas and fry them for three minutes or until they're lightly browned.
3. Remove the chickpeas with a slotted spoon and wipe the pan clean with a paper towel. Add the rest of the oil to the pan and swirl it to coat it. Add the pepper through the jalapeno to the pan and stir-fry for two more minutes.
4. Add the cumin seeds and the following five ingredients to the pan. Stir fry another thirty seconds. Add the rest of the broth and the chickpeas.
5. Bring it to a boil and remove it from the heat. Serve it over the couscous and top it with the cilantro.
6. Serve with some lemon wedges if you'd like.

Blackened Tofu Po'Boys

Serves: 4

Ingredients

- 14 Oz. Extra-Firm Tofu
- 4 Sub Rolls
- 1 Tbsp. Pepper
- 1 Tbsp. Fennel Seeds
- 2 Tsp. Thyme
- 2 Tsp. Smoked Paprika
- 2 Tsp. Dry Mustard
- 1 Tsp. Garlic Powder
- 1 Tsp. Cayenne
- 1 Tsp. Marjoram
- 1 Tsp. Sage
- 2 Tbsp. Olive Oil
- Lettuce, Shredded
- Pickle Slices
- Tomato, Sliced
- ⅓ C. Mayonnaise
- ½ Tsp Smoked Paprika
- ⅛ Tsp Cayenne
- ⅛ Tsp Garlic Powder
- Pepper

Directions

1. Remove the tofu from its package. Put it on the plate and put another plate on top of it. Then add some weight to press it down. Set it aside and check the plate and drain any water if it's necessary.
2. Toast the buns and slice them. Cook them in a dry skillet a few minutes to get them toasted.
3. Mix the dry ingredients in a bowl and cut the tofu into sixteen slices. Fill a small dish up with some water.
4. Heat the oil in a skillet and drunk a piece of tofu into the water. Then dredge it in the spice mix and pat it to cover all the sides. Once the tofu is done, put it in the hot skillet and fry until its blackened, around three minutes on either side. Remove it to a plate and repeat with the remainder of the tofu.
5. Mix the mayonnaise through the pepper together.
6. Spread some of the sauce on the bottom of the bun and add the lettuce and a few pieces of tofu. Top with the tomatoes and pickles.

Stuffed Grape Leaves

Serves: 4-5

Ingredients

- 15.2 Oz. Grape Leaves In Brine
- ⅔ C. Basmati Rice
- ½ C. Onion, Grated
- 3 Tbsp. Mint, Minced
- 3 Tbsp. Parsley, Minced
- 3 Tbsp. Lemon Juice, Divided
- 3 Tbsp. Olive Oil
- ½ Tsp Sea Salt

Directions

1. Bring a pan of water to a boil and separate the grape leaves, putting them in a large bowl. Cover them with the boiling water and allow them to soak for an hour.
2. Put the rice and a cup of water into a pan. Bring it to a boil and reduce the heat. Cover and simmer it for fifteen minutes. Remove it from the heat and set it aside.
3. Add the rice to a bowl. Stir in the onion, mint, parsley, and a tablespoon of the lemon juice. Season with salt and add a tablespoon of the oil.
4. Lay out a grape leaf flat.
5. Add a tablespoon of the filling and fold it like a burrito.
6. Put the leaves into a plastic bag and add the rest of the lemon juice and oil. Refrigerate overnight and turn every few hours.

Affordable Vegetarian Lifestyle

Book 2

Introduction

Have you had troubles finding vegan recipes that would fit your budget? There is a handful of vegan, just like you, who want to survive and yet find few solutions for their diet.

Let's face it, everywhere food installments promote non-vegan meals. Most recipes found online are quite expensive and advertise expensive products. Is there hope for vegan college students?

The best solution of course is to find recipe books that have certified vegan meals that can be cooked up with only a few dollars.

Affordable Vegetarian Lifestyle: 23 Quick Nutrition Meal Plans to Keep You Focused and Feeling Good will help you be more motivated because you will always have delicious vegan dishes ready. The ingredients will not be costly! You will be able to keep focused, because you have the greatest affordable vegan recipes. You will also be able to feel good, because the best benefit these vegetarian recipes will make your overall health increase.

Chapter 1 Vegan Breakfasts Galore

1. The Ultimate Vegan Meatball Burger

Budget: $3 per serving

Ingredients:

- 8 vegan meatballs
- ¼ cup vegan mozzarella (grated)
- ¼ cup marinara sauce
- 2 lengthwise sliced hoagie rolls

Instructions:

1. At a low measurement, preheat to broil
2. Take the meatballs and heat them. Sauce them on a stovetop or in a microwave until they are warm.
3. Put four meatballs on the hoagie rolls. Top them with half of the grated soy cheese and half of the marinara sauce. Put on an aluminum-baking sheet that is foil-lined.
4. Put the sandwiches under the broiler to make the soy cheese melted ad bread toasted. This will take about 3 minutes.

2. Your Own Cheese to Macaroni

Budget: $2.75 per serving

Ingredients:

- 3 ½ cups elbow macaroni
- 3 ½ cups boiling water
- 2 Tbsp. soy sauce
- 1 cup nutritional yeast flakes
- 1-2 tsp. salt
- 1 1/2 tsp. garlic powder
- Pinch of turmeric
- ½ cup vegan margarine
- ½ cup flour and 1/4 cup vegetable oil
- Paprika, to taste

Instructions:

1. Preheat the oven to 360 degrees F
2. Follow the instructions on the elbow macaroni pack. Drain and put aside.
3. Use a saucepan to allow margarine melting over low heat. Get the flour for whisking.
4. Turn the heat up to medium and keep whisking over the saucepan. Stop when it is bubbly and smooth. Whisk salt, garlic powder, turmeric, soy sauce, and boiling water until dissolved. If it is bubbling thick, whisk in the nutritional yeast flakes and oil.
5. Get a casserole dish. Mix the noodles and ¾ of the sauce then place it on the dish. Cover the rest of the sauce and sprinkle paprika. Bake for about 15 minutes. Broil it until it is crisp.

3. Corn Salad with Lime

Budget: $3 per serving

Ingredients:

- 2 small red bell peppers that are chopped finely (2 cups, which is about 200g)
- 2 cans of 15 ounces of rinsed and drained low sodium black beans
- 1 tablespoon pure maple syrup
- 1 chopped avocado
- 1 teaspoon chili powder
- 1 ¼ cups frozen pre-cooked corn
- ½ teaspoon ground cumin
- ¼ cup fresh lime juice (measuring up to 4 or 5 limes)
- 1/8 teaspoon fine sea salt

Instructions:

1. Preheat the oven to 400 degrees. Get 2 sheet pans and line them with parchment paper. On one pan, add the chopped bell pepper. With the salt and pepper, season it. On the other one, add corn and spread it. In the middle rack, add the bell peppers. On the bottom rack, add corn. To add firmness to the soft flavor, roast for about 10 minutes.

2. While waiting, rinse and drain the beans, then warm them.

3. Mix the limejuice, chili powder, salt, syrup, and cumin. Whisk them with effort. This will create your lime sauce. Put a small pan over the stove. The heat should be over medium-low. Cook for only a few minutes to heat through.

4. Check the oven and see if the vegetables are done. Add the vegetables in a large serving bowl. Put in the beans, pour the lime sauce, and toss. Take note to coat evenly. This will add a citrus taste to your salad. You will not have to add a lot of salt. Taste it to see if it creates a true delight. You may add seasoning or not.

5. Chop the avocado and put it in before serving. This would be good as a main dish for 2 people. As a side dish, it would be good for 4 people. It can be served warm or chilled.

4. Noodle Soup from Mexico

Budget: $3 per serving

Ingredients:

- 4-6 large tomatoes, must be cut into big cubes
- 2 tablespoons oregano
- 2 tablespoons vegetable oil
- 2 tablespoons cumin
- 1 medium white onion, must be sliced into big cubes
- 1 pack of 16 ounces angel hair pasta, broken into pieces (1 inch sized)
- 1 clove garlic
- 32 ounces of vegetable broth
- ½ tablespoon salt
- ½ tablespoon pepper

Instructions:

1. Use a blender to puree the onions, oil, tomatoes, and garlic. Put it in a large pot then cook over medium heat.
2. Add broth, salt, pepper, cumin, noodles, and oregano. You may add other spicier ingredients like jalapenos or chili flakes to make it a tastier bowl. Cook for about 12 to 15 minutes. Simmer the pot. If your noodles are tender, you are ready.
3. You may garnish cilantro, sliced avocado, and soy sour sauce as optional toppings.

5. Scramble Your Tofu

Budget: $1. 67

Ingredients:

- 1 package of drained and mashed firm tofu
- 1 minced clove garlic
- 1 tablespoon olive oil
- 1 tablespoon chopped flat-leaf parsley
- ½ teaspoon turmeric
- ½ teaspoon salt
- ½ cup of lemon juice
- ¼ cup diced green pepper
- ¼ cup diced onion

Instructions:

1. In a medium sized bowl for mixing, mix the crumbled tofu, salt, lemon juice, and turmeric.
2. Over medium heat, place a pan and add onion, pepper, and garlic. Sauté until soft.
3. Add in the pan the tofu mixture. Cook until the tofu pieces start to brown. Stir in the soy bacon pieces, parsley, and pepper as you like it best.

6. White Bean Sauce Spaghetti

Budget: $1.73 per serving

Ingredients:

- 2 minced garlic cloves
- ¼ cup vegan margarine
- 1 ½ cups of unsweetened soy milk
- 2 cups of rinsed and drained white beans
- Salt and pepper

Instructions:

1. Over low heat, put in a sauté pan have the margarine melt. Add the garlic. Allow it to cook for about 2 to 3 minutes.
2. Put the margarine mixture in a food processor like a blender. Add 1 cup of soy milk and the white beans. Blend this and ensure it is totally smooth. If you find the sauce too thick, you can add more soy milk to suit your taste.
3. Pour the sauce into the pan once more. Make the heat low. Season with salt and pepper to taste. If you like add parsley or other fresh herbs. Cook this until the sauce is warm.

7. Quesadillas with Eggs, Black Beans, and Spinach

Budget: $3 per serving

Ingredients:

- 1 can of 15 ounces rinsed black beans
- 1 ripe diced avocado
- 2 teaspoons of divided canola oil
- 4 whole wheat tortillas of 8 inches each
- 1/2 cup shredded cheese, preferably with pepper taste
- 1/2 cup divided prepared fresh salsa

Instructions:

1. In a medium sized bowl, mix the beans, cheese, and ¼ cup of the prepared salsa.
2. On your working surface, prepare your tortillas by spreading ½ cup of the mixture on half of each tortilla.
3. Fold the tortillas evenly and gently press to make them flat.
4. In a large nonstick skillet, heat 1 teaspoon of the oil at a medium temperature. Put in 2 quesadillas and turn once. Cook until the sides are golden. This will take 2 to 4 minutes.
5. Put them on a cutting board. Use a foil to keep them warm. Do this again with the rest of the quesadillas and oil. Serve with the remaining salsa and the avocado.

8. Roll-ups of Faux-Turkey and 'Cheese'

Budget: $3 per serving

Ingredients:

- 3 large tortillas
- 2 tablespoons of vegan mayonnaise
- 2 tablespoons of mustard
- 1 pack of Tofurky Deli Slices
- 1 pack of Follow Your Heart American Style Slices
- 1 spinach bunch

Instructions:

1. Create "cheese" by laying the vegan mayonnaise and mustard on the tortillas.
2. Put in the deli slices, spinach, and "cheese".
3. Lengthwise roll the tortillas tightly, cut into pieces of 2 inch size and serve. You can create 12 roll ups with this.

9. Tempeh Bacon Salad with Vegan Bleu Cheese

Budget: $3 per serving

Ingredients:

- 1 quartered head of iceberg lettuce
- 1 diced medium red onion
- 1 tablespoon apple cider vinegar
- 1 pinch black pepper
- 1/2 cup vegan mayonnaise
- 1/2 halved grape tomatoes
- 1/3 cup vegan bacon bits
- 1/4 cup plain almond milk

Instructions:

1. In a small bowl, mix the apple cider vinegar, black pepper, and vegan mayonnaise.
2. One at a time, put in a teaspoon of almond until there is consistency. Add in the vegan bleu cheese.
3. Over each lettuce wedge, pour the dressing. Sprinkle with the onions, bacon bits, and tomatoes. Do this for each salad in an equal amount.

10. An Avocado and Pumpernickel Bread Delight

Budget: $3 per serving

Ingredients:

- 2 pumpernickel bread slices
- Mustard
- 1/2 pitted, mashed, and peeled avocado
- 1/4 cup sauerkraut
- Thousand Island dressing

Instructions:

1. On one bread slice, put on some mustard. On the other, spread the Thousand Island dressing.
2. On a skillet that is lightly oiled, place the bread slices with its dry side down. Put one avocado on top of one slice. On the other slice top with the sauerkraut.
3. Grill the sandwich, over a medium heat. You would want the sandwich to be hot and light brown. This will take 5 minutes.
4. Put the sandwich halves together.

Chapter 2 Lunch Break Time

11. A Cauliflower Plate

Budget: $3 per serving

Ingredients:

Cauliflower

- 1 large head of sliced cauliflower, bite-sized florets
- Salt and freshly ground black pepper
- 2 to 3 tablespoons olive oil

Chipotle sauce

- 2 tablespoons lime juice
- 2 to 3 tablespoons adobo sauce (from a chipotle peppers can)
- ⅓ cup mayonnaise
- Salt and freshly ground black pepper, to taste

Seasoned lentils

- 2 large pressed garlic cloves
- 2 tablespoons tomato paste
- 2 cups vegetable broth or water
- 1 tablespoon olive oil
- 1 cup chopped white onion
- ½ teaspoon ground cumin
- ½ teaspoon chili powder
- ¾ cup brown lentils, picked over for debris and rinsed

Other Essentials

- 8 small, round corn tortillas
- ½ cup packed fresh cilantro leaves or fresh spring greens

Instructions:

1. For the cauliflower: Preheat oven to 425 degrees Fahrenheit. With just enough olive oil, toss cauliflower florets. Cover them with a layer of oil lightly and evenly. With salt and pepper, season it.

2. On a large baking sheet that's rimmed, set up the florets in one layer. The roasting will take 30 to 35 minutes. Toss halfway. Wait until the florets look very golden on the edges.

3. In a medium-sized pot, warm the olive oil over medium heat. For about 5 minutes, sauté the onion and garlic with just a salt dash. Make sure the onions are soft and becoming translucent.

4. Add the cumin tomato paste, and chili powder. Sauté for an additional minute, stir constantly. Put in the lentils and the vegetable broth or water.

5. Raise heat. Make the mixture simmer gently. Cook the mixture uncovered, for 20 minutes to 45 minutes. Ensure the lentils are tender and well cooked. Put the heat at minimum, if you need to keep a gentle simmer. If the liquid evaporates before lentils are finished, put in more broth or water. Once the lentils are finished drain extra liquid, then cover and put aside.

6. For the chipotle sauce, whisk all the ingredients and put aside. You can use a blender to puree everything.

7. Over medium heat, warm each tortilla in a pan individually. Stack the warm tortillas. You may cover them with a tea towel if you choose to serve later.

8. On each tortilla, top the cauliflower, lentil mixture, a chipotle sauce drizzle, and a nice chopped cilantro sprinkle.

12. Artichokes and Spinach-Oh My!

Budget: $1.34 per serving

Ingredients:

- 12 ounces fettuccine
- 8 ounces of mushrooms
- 5 cups vegetable broth
- 4 garlic cloves
- 4 ounces frozen cut spinach
- 1 can of 14 ounces artichoke hearts
- 1 medium yellow onion
- 2 tablespoons olive oil
- 1 teaspoon of dried oregano
- ½ teaspoon of fried thyme
- 15-20 cranks of freshly cracked

Instructions:

1. Rinse the mushrooms and slice thinly. Drain the artichoke hearts can and chop them roughly into pieces that are bite sized. Slice the onion and garlic thinly.

2. In a large pot, put the vegetable broth, artichoke hearts, mushrooms, olive oil, and onions. Break the fettuccine into two. Add it to the pot. Also include the oregano, thyme, and a fair amount the cranks of freshly cracked pepper. You would want to push the mixture down under the broth. Put a lid on the pot and put it over high heat and ensure a rolling boil.

3. *When it boils, stir the pot. This will distribute the ingredients evenly and avoid sticky pasta. Turn the heat down to low. Make sure the pot is simmering. Do this with a lid on for 10-15 minutes. The pasta should be tender and the liquid mostly absorbed. Stir from time to time.*

4. *Add the frozen spinach when the pasta is cooked. Let the pasta's heat to thaw the spinach. Stir the pot more. This will break spinach clumps they are melting. Serve hot.*

13. Currying Vegan Chicken Fast

Budget: $3 per serving

Ingredients:

- 1 package Lightly Seasoned Beyond Meat
- 1 cup blanched cauliflower florets
- 1 tablespoon canola oil
- 1 teaspoon minced garlic
- 1 teaspoon cracked coriander
- 1 teaspoon minced ginger
- 1.5 teaspoon paprika
- 1.5 teaspoon curry paste
- 1/2 teaspoon cumin
- 1.5 teaspoon curry powder
- 1/4 cup coconut milk
- 1 tablespoon tamari
- 2 tablespoon brown sugar
- 1 sliced onion
- 1 red sliced pepper
- 1 cup blanched broccoli florets

Instructions:

1. Get the canola oil, sauté garlic and ginger it for about 1 minute.
2. Off heat, stir in the curry paste, coriander, curry powder, cumin, and paprika
3. For about 2 minutes, cook over low heat. Stir in the brown sugar, coconut milk, and tamari. Cook until the sugar and sauce is dissolved and hot respectively. Be careful not to boil.
4. Put the sauce aside. Sauté the onions. Make them translucent. Put in peppers, broccoli, and cauliflower. Saute the ingredients.
5. Put in the Beyond Meat then sauté for 2 minutes. Stir in the curry sauce and serve with brown rice. It is best served warm.

14. Noodles from Thailand

Ingredients:

- 8 ounces whole-grain noodles
- 1 package frozen Asian-style vegetables of 12 ounces
- 3 tablespoons chopped, roasted, unsalted peanuts
- 3 tablespoons low-sodium soy sauce, or to taste
- 2 tablespoons brown rice syrup
- 2 tablespoons fresh lime juice (using 1 to 2 limes)
- 4 minced cloves garlic
- 2 1green onions, white and light green parts
- cup mung bean sprouts
- ¼ cup chopped fresh cilantro
- 1 lime, cut into wedges

Instructions:

1. Follow the directions of the noodle pack. Drain and put aside.
2. In a large saucepan, mix the soy sauce, lime juice, brown rice syrup, garlic, and ¼ cup water. Boil the mixture with medium heat. Get the Asian mixed vegetables and stir it. Ensure the vegetables are crisp but tender.
3. Add the mung bean sprouts to the cooked noodles. Toss then coat. Cook until thoroughly finished.
4. Garnish the noodles with the green onions, cilantro, lime wedges, and chopped peanuts then serve.

15. A Lebanese Rice Dish

Budget: $3 per serving

Ingredients:

- 8 ounces short grain rice
- 2½ ounces rice noodles broken into small pieces
- 150ml natural yogurt
- 1½ ounces butter
- 1 finely diced onion
- 100 grams pine nuts
- 200 ml water
- 2 crushed garlic cloves
- 1lb and 1 ounce minced lamb
- 2 teaspoon ground cumin
- 2 teaspoon ground coriander
- 2 sprigs fresh coriander
- A dash of Worcestershire sauce
- A lamb stock cube
- Salt and pepper

Instructions:

1. Sweat the onion and garlic in a heavy based frying pan. Add the lamb mince. Cook until the ingredients until it browns.

2. Put in the cumin, ground coriander, and a dash of Worcester sauce. Season it with salt and pepper.

3. For a little bit of stock, create it with the lamb stock cube. Over a high heat cook until the mince is cooked thoroughly.

4. In the melted butter, fry the rice noodles. Add the rice. For 1 minute, fry the ingredients. Add the water and cook. This should take about 20 minutes. Do this at least until the water is absorbed and the rice is tender. (You can add more boiling water if needed)

5. Chop the coriander roughly and put it on the yogurt. In a dry pan, toast the pine nuts. This should only take a minute.

6. Remove from the heat. When it is cooked, make the rice a dish for serving. With the cooked mince, top the rice dish. Drizzle the mince over the yogurt. Chop the coriander then with the toasted pine nuts, sprinkle. Serve right away.

16. Sweet Potatoes with a Treasure

Budget: $3 per serving

Ingredients:

- 1 medium baked white sweet potato
- 1/2 cup scooped potato flesh
- 1/4 teaspoon turmeric
- 1/4 teaspoon salt
- 1 teaspoon extra virgin olive oil
- 1/4 teaspoon garlic powder
- 1 teaspoon maple syrup
- Optional: nutritional yeast to taste for a cheezy accent
- Parsley to garnish

Instructions:

1. To make a sweet potato that is tender, bake in the oven. This should bake 400 degrees for 30-60 minutes.
2. Take off the top of the flaky potato skin. In order to peel the potato easily, make it crispy and light.
3. Take out the potato flesh by the scoop. Mash the potato with filling ingredients. Put the mash in the potato. Garnish and serve warm.

17. Priceless Parsley Salad

Budget: $3 per serving

Ingredients:

- 4 cups of fresh flat-leaf parsley leaves
- 1 thinly sliced large red onion
- 1 teaspoon pomegranate molasses
- ¼ cup pomegranate seeds
- 1½ teaspoon sugar
- 1 teaspoon ground sumac
- 3 tablespoons olive oil
- 1 tablespoon red wine vinegar
- Kosher salt

Instructions:

1. In a medium bowl, toss sugar, onion, and sumac. Then season the ingredients with salt. Let it sit 30 minutes.
2. Put in oil, pomegranate molasses, and vinegar. Toss the mixture to combine. Allow it to sit again for 5 minutes.
3. Toss in the parsley and pomegranate seeds before serving. Season with salt.

18. Stew with an African Taste

Budget: $2 per serving

Ingredients:

- 800g peeled sweet potato, cut into 2cm pieces
- 1 large peeled, finely chopped carrot
- 2 finely chopped celery sticks
- 1 large thinly sliced brown onion
- 400g can of diced tomatoes, no-added-salt
- 2 crushed garlic cloves
- 1 tablespoon curry powder
- 2 teaspoons olive oil
- 1/2 teaspoon caster sugar
- 250ml water
- 185ml light coconut milk
- 1 bunch trimmed English spinach, leaves coarsely chopped
- 40g roasted unsalted peanuts
- 2 cups steamed SunRice Basmati Rice, to serve

Instructions:

1. In a large saucepan, heat the oil over medium heat. Put in the onion, carrot, and celery. Stir until soft.
2. Add the curry powder and garlic. Stir until aromatic.
   Put in the sweet potato. Stir again until combined.
3. Stir in water, coconut milk, and tomato then boil. Make the heat low. Partially cover the ingredients then simmer until the sweet potato is tender. Stir in half the peanuts and sugar. Do this occasionally while cooking for 3-4 minutes to develop the flavors.
4. Stir in the spinach until it wilts. Top the bowls with remaining peanuts.

19. Your Very own Enchilada

Budget: $4 per serving

Ingredients:

Enchilada Sauce

- 2 tablespoons whole wheat flour
- 4 tablespoons chili powder
- 2 tablespoons vegetable oil
- 1 tablespoon dried oregano
- 1 tablespoon tomato paste
- 1 teaspoon garlic powder
- 2 cups vegetable broth
- 1/2 teaspoon salt

Enchilada Filling

- 8 or more corn tortillas
- 1 small zucchini
- 1/2 white onion
- 1 can black beans, drained
- 1 bell pepper
- Salt and black pepper
- 1/4 cup sliced olives
- 1/2 cup chopped cilantro
- 3 green onions

Instructions:

Part One

1. Heat 2 tablespoons of vegetable oil in a small saucepan, until warm.
2. In a pan, put in 2 tablespoons of flour. Whisk until there are no clumps.
3. Add the chili powder, garlic powder, salt, oregano, and the tomato paste slowly. Combine and whisk.
4. Also slowly pour in the vegetable broth, in thirds. Whisk to unite the spices and have no lumps.

5. Lower the heat and allow simmering for 15 minutes. Adjust spices if needed.

Part Two

1. Chop one white onion half. Put it in a skillet. Add a splash of water and let it to cook to soften.

2. While cooking chop 1 bell pepper and 1 small zucchini squash loosely. Make them bite-sized pieces. Put them into the pan.

3. With a few pinches of salt and pepper season it. Let it cook until fully softened.

4. Add the drained black beans into the pan until warmed. Then take it away from the heat.

5. Chop the black olives and the cilantro. Slice the green onions.

Part Three

1. Preheat the oven to 350°. Along a large casserole dish's bottom, spread 1/2 cup of the enchilada sauce.

2. Put it in the microwave, then heat the tortillas for 30 seconds.

3. Pour a lot of sauce into a skillet that is not heated. Dip one side into the sauce. Coat both sides by flipping.

4. Add 2-3 tablespoons of the vegetables and black beans. Put in a few olives, green onions, and cilantro sprinkling.

5. Roll the enchilada gently around the filling. Place it into the casserole dish. Ensure the seam is towards the bottom.

6. Cover the dish with foil. Bake at 350° for about 20 minutes.

20. A Veggie Bread Pudding

Budget: $3 per serving

Ingredients:

- 100g dairy-free margarine
- 1 large pinch of ground ginger
- 10 thick slices of quality stale bread
- 1 large pinch of ground cinnamon
- 100g sultanas
- 1 zest of orange
- 100g apricots
- 5 tablespoons quality thick-cut marmalade

Custard:

- 1 vanilla pod
- 6 tablespoons golden caster sugar
- 800ml unsweetened organic soya milk
- 5 tablespoons corn flour

Instructions:

1. Preheat the oven to 180 degrees. In a bowl, combine the margarine, cinnamon, orange zest, and ginger. On the bread, spread the rest of margarine.
2. Diagonally cut the bread. In a single layer, place roughly a third. Also chop the apricots roughly. Scatter a third portion into the dish with a third of the sultanas.
3. With another layer of bread, cover. Scatter more dried fruit and cover with the rest of the bread. Put aside.
4. For the custard, split the vanilla pod by its length and scrape out the seeds. In a medium pan, put the seeds with the rest of the custard ingredients and 400ml of water. Whisk until smooth and well mixed. Put over a medium–low heat. Gently simmer until the custard is almost boiling.
5. Pour the custard over the bread. On top, scatter the rest of the dried fruit. Allow it to soak for about 20 minutes. Put in the hot oven until lightly golden.

6. While waiting, in a pan warm the marmalade over a low heat. Take the pudding and brush it over with the warm marmalade. Put it back in the oven for until golden. Let it slightly cool then tuck in.

Chapter 3 Dinner Must Haves 21. Roasted

Squash with Spices

Budget: $2 per serving

Ingredients: 1 butternut squash

- ground coriander seeds
- olive oil
- ground fennel
- red chilli flakes
- ground cumin
- nutmeg & cinnamon

Instructions:

1. Preheat oven to 200°C. Cut the squash in half lengthwise and take out the seeds. Peel and slice into wedges that are portion sized.
2. With olive oil, smear all cut sides. Put in the sea salt and black pepper. Scatter the spices.
3. For about 30 minutes, bake in the oven. Ensure the squash is tender and caramelized slightly.

22. Kale Salad with Pecans and Apple

Budget: $3 per serving

Ingredients:

- 8 ounces kale
- ½ cup pecans
- 1 medium Granny Smith apple
- 1½ tablespoons apple cider vinegar
- 4 to 5 medium radishes
- 2 ounces soft chilled goat cheese
- ½ cup dried cranberries

Dressing

- 1½ teaspoons honey
- 3 tablespoons olive oil
- 1 tablespoon smooth Dijon mustard
- Sea salt and freshly ground pepper, to taste

Instructions:

1. Preheat the oven to 350 degree. On a baking tray, spread the pecans. Toast them until light golden for about 5 to 10 minutes. Tossing the pecans and bake evenly. Take the tray from the oven and put aside.

2. Take the kale leaves off from the stems. Chop the kale into bite-sized pieces with a chef's knife. Put the kale in a big salad bowl. Add a pinch of sea salt over the kale. With your hands, massage the leaves lightly. Do this with big handfuls until the leaves are darker.

3. Slice the radishes thinly then put them with the rest of the ingredients in the bowl.

4. Chop the pecans and cranberries coarsely. Include them in the bowl. Chop the apple into bite-sized pieces then also add to the bowl. Crumble the goat cheese.

5. Whisk the dressing ingredients in a small bowl together. Pour the dressing over the salad. Toss until evenly coated. Serve immediately or marinate 10-20 minutes before serving.

23. Soup Bowl of Lentil-Veggies

Budget: $5 per serving

Ingredients:

- 2 tablespoon olive oil
- 3-4 carrots
- 2 garlic cloves
- 1 can of 15 ounces black beans
- 1 medium onion
- 3 ribs celery
- 1 teaspoon cumin
- 1 cup brown lentils
- ¼ teaspoon cayenne pepper
- 1 teaspoon oregano
- ½ teaspoon smoked paprika
- Freshly ground black pepper
- ½ teaspoon salt
- 1 can of 15 ounces petite-diced tomatoes
- 4 cups vegetable broth

Instructions:

1. Dice the onion and mince the garlic. In a large pot, cook both with olive oil over medium heat. Ensure the ingredients are tender.
2. While waiting, slice the celery. Peel and slice the carrots. Put the celery and carrots to the pot. For about 5 more minutes, saute.
3. Drain the black beans and put them in the pot. Dry lentils, smoked paprika, cumin, cayenne pepper, oregano, and some freshly cracked pepper.
4. Put in the diced tomatoes and the juices. Also add the vegetable broth, and stir to mix.
5. Turn up the heat to medium high. Let the pot boil. Turn the heat down to low, put on the lid, and simmer for half an hour. Ensure the lentils are tender.
6. Taste the soup and add salt if necessary. Serve hot.

Vegetarian

Table of Contents

Book 3

Chapter 1: Sweets And Snack Options 2

Chapter 2: Week One 7

Chapter 3: Week Two 10

Chapter 4: Week Three 13

Chapter 5: Week Four 16

Chapter 6: Week Five 19

Chapter 7: Week Six 22

Chapter 8: Week Seven 26

Chapter 9: Week Eight 30

Chapter 10: Week Nine 33

BOOK 4

Introduction 37

Chapter 1: Vegetarian Breakfast Recipes 39

Chapter 2: Vegetarian Lunch Recipes 44

Chapter 3: Vegetarian Dinner Recipes 50

Chapter 4: Vegetarian Smoothie, Shakes and Juice Recipes 58

Chapter 5: Vegetarian Dessert Recipes 66

Book 3

Chapter 1: Sweets And Snack Options

In this chapter you will be introduced to some great Vegetarian snacks. These snack options range from sweet to savoury, so there is something for whatever you are craving. Many of these snack options also allow room for you to add your own twist. You can add different fruits, vegetables or seasonings to make them more appealing to you.

Vegan 'Yogurt'

Ingredients:

- Coconut milk- 28 ounces
- Agar Agar- 1-tablespoon
- Sugar Or Maple Syrup- 2 tablespoons
- Probiotic Capsules- 4

Instructions:

Add shaken coconut milk to a pan. Whisk smooth. Sprinkle Agar Agar onto the coconut milk. Simmer this mix. Turn the heat to low, and cook 10 minutes, whisking occasionally, until the Agar Agar has completely dissolved.

Cool until this is just warm to the touch. Add the ingredients from 4 probiotic capsules. Whisk and taste.

Add up sugar or maple syrup.

Pour the yogurt into canning jars fresh from the dishwasher. Using fresh lids, cap each jar, and place in the oven for 24 hours with the light on for warmth. Do not disturb! Chill the yogurt for 6 hours, checking to make sure it has not separated. If so, stir well, and use that jar first.

Greek Style Quick Yogurt

Ingredients:

- Coconut Meat- 2 cups
- Coconut Water- ½ cup
- Probiotic Capsules- 4
- Pink sea salt- just a bit
- Feel free to add Carrots, Apples, Bananas, or any other small fruit of your choosing

Instructions:

Blend 2 cups young coconut meat, ½ cup coconut water, the ingredients from 4 probiotic capsules, and a bit of pink sea salt. Blend, starting on low, and slowly increasing, until the mixture is super-smooth. Sweeten to taste. Place in container and refrigerate at least two hours.

Chips And Salsa

Ingredients:

- Large Beefsteak Tomatoes- 4
- Jalapeno- ½
- Scallions- 3
- Cilantro- a handful

Instructions:

Coarse chop 4 large beefsteak tomatoes. Mix ½ jalapeno (seeded and chopped), 3 scallions and a handful of cilantro in a bowl. Layer these, or add in garlic, pineapple, watermelon, zucchini, green pepper, strawberries, or what you enjoy. Serve with pita, corn, or tofu chips.

Toast With Fruit Butter

Ingredients:

- Seasonal Fruit
- Sugar- 1 cup per pint of fruit
- Fruit Pectin- 1 package per 4 pints of fruit
- Lemon Juice
- Spices of your choice

Instructions:

Place three small plates in the freezer. Using your slow cooker, take seasonal fruit, a bit of sugar (1 cup per pint), fruit pectin (one packet for every 4 pints), and lemon juice; plus any spices that you would enjoy. On low, stir at 1 hour, then at the 2-hour mark. Cover, raise to high, and cook 2-3 hours. Test a spoonful of jam by seeing if it becomes firm on a plate from the freezer. If not, cook a while longer.

Muffin Square

Ingredients:

- Ripe Bananas- 2 large
- Vanilla- 1 tsp (optional)
- Rolled Oats- 2 cups
- Salt- ½ tsp (optional)
- Dried Dates- ¼ cup
- Chopped Nuts- ¼ cup

Instructions:

Peel and mash 2 large, very ripe bananas, until there are no large chunks left. Add 1 teaspoon vanilla (optional), 2 cups rolled oats, 1/2 teaspoon salt (optional), 1/4 cup pitted, chopped dried dates, and 1/4 cup chopped nuts — such as walnuts, hazelnuts, or pecans, stirring well after each addition.

Pat into a well-oiled 9 x 9 pan, and bake in a 350 degree oven for 30 minutes, or until the edges begin to crisp. Place the pan on a wire rack, and cut into bars when mostly cool.

Chapter 2: Week One

Day 1:

Breakfast: Mango/orange/beet juice smoothie

Noon Meal: Southwest Salad-greens with black beans, corn and peppers

Evening Meal: Sun-dried tomatoes, Spinach, and Tofu <u>Quiche</u> (save some for later)

Sun-Dried Tomatoes, Spinach, And Tofu <u>Quiche</u>

Ingredients:

- Ground Flax
- Water
- Almond Flour
- Dried Parsley
- Dried Oregano
- Kosher Salt
- Drained Tofu
- Garlic Cloves
- Mushrooms
- Fresh Chives
- Basil Leaves
- Sun-Dried Tomatoes
- Baby Spinach
- Nutritional Yeast
- Sea Salt
- Black And Rep Pepper

Instructions:

Whisk 1 tablespoon ground flax and 3 tablespoons water. Set aside to let gel.

Stir together 1 cup almond flour, 1 cup oat flour, 1 teaspoon dried parsley, 1 teaspoon dried oregano, and 1/2 tsp. kosher salt. Add the gelled flax mixture, and some water (no more than 3 tablespoons) until it is stick together when pressed between your fingers.

Working from the centre, press into a crust to the top of the rim of an oiled pan. Poke a few holes with a fork so air can escape, and bake at 350 degrees for 13-15 minutes.

Meanwhile, break apart and blend 14 ounces pressed and drained tofu until creamy. Add a bit of almond mix if needed. In a skillet, sauté 1 thin sliced leek and 3 minced garlic cloves. Once tender add 8-oz sliced mushrooms, and cook until most of the moisture is go- about 10 minutes. Add 1/2 cup chopped fresh chives, 1/2 cup chopped fresh basil leaves, 1/3 cup chopped oil-packed sun-dried tomatoes, 1-cup baby spinach, 2 tbsp. nutritional yeast, 1 teaspoon dried oregano, 3/4-1 teaspoon fine grain sea salt. And black and rep pepper, to taste, Cook until the spinach is completely wilted.

Remove from heat, and add the tofu mixture. Stir until completely combined. Spoon into baked crust, and bake at 375 degrees for 30-40 minutes, until the top of the quiche is done. Cool 20 minutes on a baking rack for the easiest cutting.

Day 2:

Breakfast: Oats or other cereal and fruit

Noon Meal: Fresh spring mix with leftovers from last night

Evening Meal: Baked Ziti with vegetables

Day 3:

Breakfast: Overnight oats with fresh or canned fruits

Noon Meal: Tostada

Tostadas

Ingredients:

- Corn Tortillas
- Broth
- Chopped Onion
- Minced Garlic
- Black Beans
- Lemon
- Cumin
- Green Chillies
- Salt And Pepper

Instructions:

Toast 8 good-quality corn tortillas in the oven, or individually in a pan, until brown and crunchy.

Heat 3 tablespoons broth, or 1 tablespoon oil, and sauté 1 medium chopped onion and 2 cloves minced garlic about 5 minutes, or until golden. Add ¼ cup water, 2 15 cans of drained, rinsed black beans (use your own if you have them), the juice of ½ lemon, 2 teaspoons cumin, and 2 small seeded and sliced hot green chillies (optional). Salt and pepper to taste. Mash, and remove from heat.

Spread tortillas with a generous serving of the bean mixture, and top with greens, tomatoes, corn, avocados, cashew cream, and salsa.

Evening Meal: Quiche, and a fresh salad

Day 4:

Breakfast: Fresh fruit

Noon Meal: Creamy soup- tomato, cauliflower, or mushroom

Evening Meal: Mexican Black Bean 'Pizza'

Day 5:

Breakfast: Cereal with peaches, cinnamon, and walnuts

Noon Meal: Quiche from Day 2

Evening Meal: Hearty Roasted Vegetables

Hearty Roasted Vegetables

Ingredients:

- Brussels Sprouts
- Cauliflower
- Hard-Shell Squash
- Button Mushrooms
- Small Onions
- Honey-Balsamic Vinegar-Garlic Mix
- Salt And Pepper

Instructions:
Start with 8 oz. of Brussels sprouts, halved. Keeping this as an average size, break apart 1 cauliflower, and cut up 2 hard-shell squash (acorn is a good choice) into cubes about the same size. Add 12 oz. button mushrooms and two small onions quartered. Mix well, and place on lined cookie sheets. Bake at 350 degrees for 20 to 30 minutes, turning once halfway through. Baste the vegetables with a honey-balsamic vinegar-garlic mix, and season with salt and pepper and other spices if desired. Roast 5 more minutes, turn once again, and baste the vegetables again.

Chapter 3: Week Two

Day 1:

Breakfast: Muffin Squares

Noon Meal: Southwest Wrap of tofu, leftover pasta bake or chickpeas; spring mix; and a spicy dressing in a whole-wheat tortilla

Evening Meal: Pasta and Portobello mushrooms with extra soup or vodka sauce

Day 2:

Breakfast: Jelly-filled muffins

Jelly-Filled Muffins

Ingredients:

- All-Purpose Flour
- Baking Powder
- Baking Soda
- Ground Nutmeg
- Fine Salt
- Soy Or Rice Milk
- Granulated Sugar
- Vegetable Oil
- Vanilla Extract
- Muffin Cups With Paper Liners

Instructions:

In a large bowl, sift together 1 1/2 cups all-purpose flour, 3/4-teaspoon baking powder, 1/2-teaspoon baking soda, 1/2-teaspoon ground nutmeg, 1/2-teaspoon fine salt. Set aside.

In a glass or plastic bowl, mix 1-cup plain soy or rice milk, 1-teaspoon cider vinegar, and 2 tablespoons cornstarch. Mix until the cornstarch has dissolved. Make a well in the dry ingredients, and pour the milk mixture into the well. Stir well, adding 3/4 cup plus 2 tablespoons granulated sugar, 1/3-cup vegetable oil, and 2 teaspoons vanilla extract. There will be a few lumps in the mixture.

Line the full-sized muffin cups with paper liners, and fill each one about ¾ full. Using a spoon, put a small indentation in the batter, and fills each with 1 heaping teaspoon of raspberry, strawberry, or grape jam or preserves. Bake in a 350-degree oven for about 20-25 minutes, until the tops of the muffins are firm. Remove from pan, and cool completely on a wire rack.

Noon Meal: Vegan Mac and cheese- add fruit salad for a full meal

Evening Meal: Three-bean chilli and Pesto

Day 3:

Breakfast: Cereal and fruit

Noon Meal: Wrap Day: rice, beans and greens

Evening Meal: Shepard's pie- make extra of the vegetable stew to use for lunch

Day 4:

Breakfast: Apple/peach/kale smoothie

Noon Meal: Vegetable stew

Evening Meal: Baked Lasagna Rolls

Baked Lasagna Rolls

Ingredients:

- Eggplants
- Salt
- Whole-Wheat Lasagna Noodles
- Tofu 'Cheese'
- Tomato Sauce

Instructions:

Slice 2 eggplants into ¼ inch strips lengthwise, salt and place in a colander in the sink to drain and shed bitterness. Then rinse, place on kitchen towel, and use a weighted cookie sheet to remove excess water. Then bake for 13-15 minutes in a 425-degree oven, turning oven down to 375 once eggplant is done. Set aside or use cooked whole-wheat lasagna noodles.

Make the tofu 'cheese': 2 lemons, juiced (~1/3 cup), 1 12-ounce block extra firm tofu, drained and pressed dry for 10 minutes. 3 Tbsp. nutritional yeast, 1/2 cup fresh basil, finely chopped, 1 Tbsp. dried oregano, 3-4 Tbsp. extra virgin olive oil, and salt and pepper to taste. Pulse in a food processor or blender, scraping when needed, until there are only small bits of basil showing.

Pour tomato sauce into the bottom of a baking dish, reserving some for topping. Scoop a generous amount of the tofu cheese mixture onto the slices/noodles, and roll up. Place each roll seam-side down in the tomato sauce. Add additional sauce on top of the rolls if wished. Bake 15-30 minutes, until the rolls are lightly browned.

Day 5:

Breakfast: Fruit salad

Noon Meal: Pita Pizzas

Evening Meal: Tangiers of apricots, couscous and chickpeas

Tangiers Of Apricots, Couscous And Chickpeas

Less a recipe than a cooking style, this is a method of a loosely covered pot, with all the ingredients cooking down and absorbing the flavours of the stock and each other.

Chapter 4: Week Three

Day 1:

Breakfast: Citrus-Granola Parfait

Citrus-Granola Parfait

Ingredients:

- Nuts
- Dried Coconut
- Zests Of A Lemon
- Orange
- Maple Syrup
- Vanilla Extract
- Top Soy Or Other Yogurts
- Cereal

Instructions:

Use seeds, nuts, dried coconut, plus the zests of a lemon, a lime, and an orange. Use the juices, some maple syrup, and vanilla extract to the mix, and stir in oats. Blend well, and dry in a 300-degree oven for 15 minutes, stir, and bake another 15 minutes. Cool completely, and use to top soy or other yogurts, or add a bit of unexpected crunch to your morning cereal.

Noon Meal: Vegan Sushi rolls- a great calcium boost!

Evening Meal: Portobello Marsala

Day 2:

Breakfast: Oats with almond milk and fresh fruit

Noon Meal: White Bean and Avocado Club sandwich

White Bean And Avocado Club Sandwich

Ingredients:

- Bread
- White Bean Paste
- Leaf Lettuce, Or Basil Leaves
- Avocado Slices
- Onion

Instructions:

Using your favourite bread, spread white bean paste on one, top with a second slice of bread, or leaf lettuce, or basil leaves. Add avocado slices, onion, or other topping, and top with bread. Bring lots of napkins!

Evening Meal: Quiche with Chard and chickpeas

Day 3:

Breakfast: Jelly-filled Muffins

Noon Meal: Pasta and pesto

Evening Meal: Peanut-Squash Stew and a fresh salad

Day 4:

Breakfast: Breakfast Toast

Breakfast Toast

This is simple, and quick. Toast your favorite bread, and spread it with refried beans. Top with avocados and onions; greens, tomatoes, and seeds, or any other combination that your taste buds enjoy!

Noon Meal: Twice-Baked Potato Boats

Twice-Baked Potato Boats

Ingredients:

- Potatoes
- Vegan Sour Cream
- Corn
- Black Bean
- Pinto Beans
- Celery
- Vegan Cheese

Instructions:

Bake 6 potatoes at 350 degrees until soft. Remove from oven and cool. Scoop out the potato flesh, leaving about a ¼ inch all around for stability. Place the scooped potatoes into a pan, and add a small amount of stock and continue cooking them. Mash well.

Stir in vegan sour cream, corn, black bean, pinto beans, celery, vegan cheese, or other toppings. Refill potato boats, heaping a bit. Return to the oven, and bake until topping is golden brown, about 15-20 minutes.

Evening Meal: Eggplant with tomatoes and basil

Day 5:

Breakfast: Cereal and fresh/frozen fruit

Noon Meal: Jackfruit in BBQ sauce, on rolls

Evening Meal: Texas-style 'Chilli' (use eggplant instead of meat), salad with leafy greens and avocado-cilantro dressing.

Chapter 5: Week Four

Day 1:

Breakfast: Muffin Squares

Noon Meal: Pita salad with dressing

Evening Meal: Potato Gnocchi With Vodka Sauce

Potato Gnocchi With Vodka Sauce

Ingredients:

- Mashed Potato
- Salt And Pepper
- Flour

Instructions:

Mix left-over mashed potato (the drier the better) or the flesh of two or three baked potatoes, mashed without milk or butter, a bit of salt and pepper and a few tablespoons of flour. Turn onto a board, and knead. The more you work this, the more flour you will require from the moisture of the potatoes. Work until this is dry enough to separate into 4 sections, and form a long roll from each section.

Use a sharp knife to cut these into pieces, and roll them individually in flour. If the touch, they are likely to stick together.

Bring a large pan of water or stock to a boil, and drop a few of these in at a time. They will sink, and then rise to the surface when they are done. Remove and toss with a small amount of oil to stop them from sticking together. Serve with sauce, and enjoy.

Day 2:

Breakfast: overnight oats

Noon Meal: Beans and Greens

Beans And Greens

Ingredients:

- Vegetable Broth
- Onion
- Bell Pepper
- Black Beans
- Rice
- Soy Sauce

- Swiss Chard
- Tomato Sauce
- Red Chilli Powder
- Nutritional Yeast
- Salt
- Ground Seeds

Instructions:

In a large pan with a tight-fitting lid, warm the vegetable broth, then add onion and bell pepper. Once these are tender, add 1-cup pre-cooked black beans, ½ cup pre-cooked rice, and 2 tablespoons soy sauce. Once these are warm, lower the heat, and add 3-4 cups Swiss chard or other greens, and cover tightly until the greens have wilted. Once the wilting is complete, add tomato sauce, a dash of red chilli powder, nutritional yeast, and salt to taste. Top with 1-2 tablespoons ground seeds, and completely warm before serving.

Evening Meal: Taco Bowls with Tempeh

Day 3:

Breakfast: Smoothie

Noon Meal: Risotto Cakes with marina

Evening Meal: Asparagus and Lemon Risotto (fry extra in cakes for lunch)

Asparagus And Lemon Risotto

Ingredients:

- Asparagus
- Vegetable Stock
- Olive Oil
- Rice
- Lemon
- Tarragon

Instructions:

Blanch 6 stalks of asparagus for 2 minutes: it will be crunchy. Set in ice water until cool. Take the tips off, and either shaves the stalks for garnish or save for use later. If you use canned asparagus, skip this step.

Warm 1-quart vegetable stock, and in a separate, deep pan, warm ta bit of olive oil, and coat 1 cup of rice until it is evenly shiny. Add about 1/3 of a cup of the stock at a time to the rice until the stock is gone, stirring constantly to avoid burning or sticking.

Set aside any extra you may have made, and add the juice of 2 lemons and the asparagus tips. Taste, and season with tarragon.

Day 4:

Breakfast: Cereal with almond milk and fruit

Noon Meal: Wheat-protein "French Dip"

Wheat-Protein "French Dip"

Cut Seitan into strips, and fry in oil. Place on a crusty roll. Serve with vegetable stock -adding a drop of liquid smoke for flavor- and Dijon-style mustard.

Evening Meal: Seven-layer Pie

Day 5:

Breakfast: Jelly Muffin

Noon Meal: Hard-shell squash with apples, meat substitute, and bread cubes

Evening Meal: One-pot Meal with Pasta

One-Pot Meal With Pasta

This recipe uses pasta, vegetables, greens, and sauces to ease cooking times. For the south-western version of this dish, use corn (fire roasted if you have it in season), cilantro, black and pinto beans, fresh onion, chili powder, cumin and pasta to make a quick, simple dish.

Chapter 6: Week Five

Day 1:

Breakfast: Overnight oats with tropical fruits

Noon Meal: Hummus, carrots and celery

Evening Meal: Cauliflower-rice stir-fry

Day 2:

Breakfast: Lentils and onions in a tomato sauce- a traditional breakfast

Noon Meal: Steamed vegetables with Garlic sauce

Steamed Vegetables With Garlic Sauce

Ingredients:

- Garlic Cloves
- Shallots
- Sea Salt
- Black Pepper
- Cornstarch
- Vegetable Stock

Instructions:

Sauté 8 garlic cloves and 2 shallots in olive oil, seasoning with a touch of sea salt and black pepper. Cook until soft. Very slowly, add up to 4 teaspoons cornstarch, then 1-cup vegetable stock, whisking well between additions to avoid lumps.

Evening Meal: Pineapple and Cashews, stir-fried

Day 3:

Breakfast: Quinoa, apple and carrot porridge

Noon Meal: Wheat berry Salad

Wheat Berry Salad

Ingredients:

- Wheat Berries
- Pan-Toast Nuts
- Celery
- Dried Fruits
- Herbs
- Lemon Juice

- Olive Oil
- Salt
- Pepper

Instructions:

Cook 1 ½ cups hard wheat berries in enough water to cover for about an hour, set aside. Pan-toast nuts, and add them to celery, dried fruits, and herbs. Once the wheat berries are cool, add them to the other ingredients. Taste and add lemon juice, olive oil, salt, or fresh pepper as desired.

Evening Meal: Spring mix topped with shredded Carrot and Avocado

Day 4:

Breakfast: Vegetable-based smoothie

Noon Meal: Orange-ginger Tofu with broccoli

Evening Meal: Mushroom Brown Rice with ginger

Day 5:

Breakfast: Lemon-Baked Tofu With Vegan Yogurt

Lemon-Baked Tofu With Vegan Yogurt

Ingredients:

- Extra Firm Tofu
- Lemon Juice
- Balsamic Vinegar
- Soy Sauce
- Lemon Zest
- Olive Oil

Instructions:

Slice 1 lb. extra firm tofu (drained and pressed) that has been sliced into ½ inch slices, and pour over a marinate of 5 tablespoons lemon juice, 1 teaspoon balsamic vinegar, 1 tablespoon soy sauce, 1teaspoon lemon zest, and 1 tablespoon olive oil that has been mixed well. Let marinate for 30 minutes, turning once. Bake 20-30 minutes at 350 degrees.

Noon Meal: Mushroom Stroganoff

Coconut-Vegetable Rice

Ingredients:

- Jasmine Rice
- Coconut Milk
- Cilantro
- Lime Juice
- Mushrooms
- Olive Oil
- Zucchini
- Red Pepper
- Minced Garlic
- Fresh Ginger
- Frozen Edamame
- Scallions Sliced

Instructions:

Steam 1 cup jasmine rice in a rice cooker with ¾ cup of coconut milk and 1 ¼ water. When complete, add 1-cup cilantro and the juice of 2 limes.

While cooking, in a large pan, sauté 8 oz. sliced mushrooms in 2 tablespoons olive oil until tender, Add 2 small sliced zucchini, 1 diced red pepper, 2 cloves minced garlic, and a tablespoon of fresh ginger. Cook for another minute.

Add to this a bit more coconut milk, ½ c frozen edamame, and 2 scallions sliced. Season to taste, and serve over the jasmine rice.

Chapter 7: Week Six

Day 1:

Breakfast: Breakfast toast

Noon Meal: Steam sugar snap peas and carrots, toss with balsamic and noodles

Evening Meal: Butternut Squash tortellini with pesto

Day 2:

Breakfast: Peach/orange smoothie

Noon Meal: Black-Bean Burger

Evening Meal: **Ratatouille**

Ingredients:

- Bell Peppers
- Soy Sauce
- Balsamic Vinegar
- Agave Nectar
- Japanese Eggplants
- Yellow Squash
- Zucchini
- Onion
- Tomatoes
- Garlic

Instructions:

Place bell peppers (red or yellow for color) onto a foil-lined cookie sheet and broil turning every 3-5 minutes until there is char on all sides. Place the peppers in a bowl and cover with plastic wrap for 5 minutes. Meanwhile, mix 2 tablespoons soy sauce, 2 tablespoons balsamic vinegar, and 2 tablespoons agave nectar in a bowl or gallon bag, mixing well. Turn down the oven to 400 degrees.

Cut 2 small Japanese eggplants, 2 small yellow squash, 1 small zucchini into ¼ to ½ inch cubes. Cut a small onion into eights, and add all the vegetables to the marinate, tossing lightly. Let the marinate rest for at least 5 minutes. Peel the skin, seeds and stems from the bell peppers, reserving any juice. Dice the peppers into ½ inch cubes, and place in the bowl with the reserved juices.

Cut 4 tomatoes in half horizontally, and scoop out most of the seeds with a knife or small spoon. Place on a parchment covered baking sheet. Place a garlic clove into the seed cavity of each tomato so the garlic does not burn.

Sprinkle lightly with rosemary. Spread the vegetables from the marinate onto the rest of the sheet, and bake for 30 minutes, turning the cubed vegetables halfway through. Baste with the remaining marinate if they look dry.

Set the cubed vegetable into the bowl with the peppers, and place the tomato halves into a pan. The skins should slide off, once they are removed, mash the tomato flesh and the garlic. Once the tomatoes have reduced, add to the other vegetables, and serve over rice or pasta.

Day 3:

Breakfast: Baked Doughnuts With Fruit

Baked Doughnuts With Fruit

Ingredients:

- Vegan Sugar
- Unsweetened Applesauce
- Plant Milk
- Grape Seed Oil
- Vanilla
- Flour
- Baking Powder
- Baking Soda
- Fresh Fruit

Instructions:

In a large bowl, mix ½ c vegan sugar, ½ c unsweetened applesauce, 1 c plant milk, plus 1 tablespoon, 2 tablespoons grape seed oil and 2 teaspoons vanilla until well-blended. Gradually, add 2 cups flour, 1-teaspoon baking powder and ½ teaspoon of baking soda, and ½ teaspoon total of spices that blend with your fruit. Gently fold in 1-cup fresh fruit.

Oil the doughnut pan, and fill each section about ¾ full. Bake at 325 for about 15 minutes, or until the tops brown. Cool completely before removing from the pan.

Noon Meal: Pita "Gyros", tofu or tempeh instead of meat

Evening Meal: Chickpea tempura-coated vegetables

Day 4:

Breakfast: Cereal with fresh fruit

Noon Meal: Fruit salad on greens

> *Evening Meal: Roasted sweet potatoes with pinto/black bean burritos*

Roasted Sweet Potatoes With Pinto/Black Bean Burritos

Ingredients:

- Sweet Potatoes
- Chickpeas
- Olive Oil
- Cumin
- Coriander
- Cinnamon
- Smoked (Or Regular) Paprika
- Salt Or Lemon Juice
- Sauce Of Hummus
- Garlic And Spices

Instructions:

Scrub and halve 4 medium sweet potatoes.

In a bowl, mix a15-ounce can chickpeas, 1/2 Tbsp. olive oil, and 1/2 tsp. each cumin, coriander, cinnamon, smoked (or regular) paprika. Taste, and a bit of salt or lemon juice if needed.

Place the sweet potatoes cut-side down on a foil-lined baking dish. Add the chickpea mixture, and bake at 400 degrees for about 20-25 minutes, or until tender.

Make a simple sauce of hummus, lemon juice, garlic and spices to top these.

Day 5:

Breakfast: Chocolate Nut Butter on toast

Noon Meal: Pot Pie

Greek-Style Caponata

Ingredients:

- Diced Tomatoes
- Zucchini
- Summer Squash
- Tomatoes Cut Into Wedges
- Large Japanese Eggplant
- Red Onion
- Potato
- Minced Garlic
- Olive Oil
- Salt
- Pepper And Oregano

Instructions:

Into a casserole dish, pour 1 14 or 15 ounce can of diced tomatoes and their juices, and spread to cover the bottom of the pan. In a bowl, combine 2 sliced zucchini, 2 summer squash, 2 tomatoes cut into wedges, a large Japanese eggplant, cut into 1 inch rounds, a red onion cut into wedges, 1 potato, cut into 1 inch cubes, 3 cloves of minced garlic, ¼ cup olive oil, and salt, pepper and oregano to taste. Pour the vegetable mixture over the tomatoes, and bake in a 400 degree oven for 30 minutes covered with foil, then about 40 minutes uncovered, or until the vegetables are golden.

Chapter 8: Week Seven

Day 1:

Breakfast: Chickpea Pancake With Seasonal Fruits

Chickpea Pancake With Seasonal Fruits

Ingredients:

- Green Onion
- Bell Peppers
- Chickpea Flour
- Garlic Powder
- Finely Ground Sea Salt
- Finely Ground Black Pepper
- Baking Powder
- Red Pepper Flakes
  Mushrooms, Cashew Cream, Avocados, Hummus Or Salsa
- For Topping

Instructions:

Finely chop 1 green onion, ¼ cup bell peppers. Mix ½ cup chickpea flour, ¼ garlic powder, ¼ teaspoon finely ground sea salt, 1/8 teaspoon finely ground black pepper, and ¼ teaspoon baking powder. Add a pinch of red pepper flakes if you wish. Mix well, adding in ½ cup water- a bit more may be needed.

In a well-oiled pan, pour one or two pancakes. These cook more slowly than traditional pancakes, and need spread out. Turn when you can slide a spatula completely under the pancake. Cook for a similar amount of time on the other side. Top with mushrooms, cashew cream, avocados, hummus or salsa.

Noon Meal: Rice Noodles and vegetables, garnished with mandarin oranges

Evening Meal: Baked Spaghetti Squash with fresh pepper, oil and vegan cheese

Day 2:

Breakfast: Baked Doughnuts

Noon Meal: Steamed Tofu-Vegetable Pot Stickers With Peanut Sauce

Steamed Tofu-Vegetable Pot Stickers With Peanut Sauce

Ingredients:

- Minced Garlic Clove
- Fresh Ginger
- Pressed Tofu
- Chopped Scallion
- Tofu Mixture

Instructions:

In a skillet, sauté 1 minced garlic clove and ½ teaspoon fresh ginger for about a minute. Crumble and sauté 8 ounces drained and pressed tofu for about 5 minutes more. Add one chopped scallion, and remove from heat.

Place the won ton wrapper in a diamond shape in front of you. Put 1 teaspoon of the tofu mixture in the center of the wrapper and moisten the upper diamond edges. Fold the bottom up, then each side in to meet the bottom corner (looks like an envelope). Fold the top down, and seal with the edges. Place seam side down in a bamboo steamer. Leave room between these! Steam for 5 minutes until the outer surface is shiny and a few bubbles form.

Evening Meal: Chard and Chickpea with pasta

Day 3:

Breakfast: Jelly Muffins

Noon Meal: Portobello 'burgers' with all the trimmings

Evening Meal: Pine Nut Sauce On Rice

Pine Nut Sauce On Rice

Ingredients:

- Grape Or Cherry Tomatoes
- Kalamata Olives
- Minced Garlic Cloves

- Olive Oil
- Fresh Lemon Juice
- Balsamic Vinegar
- Sea Salt
- Black Pepper
- Pine Nuts
- Fresh Basil

Instructions:

Halve 2 1/2 cups grape or cherry tomatoes, and place in a giant bowl. Add 1/2 cup kalamata olives, pitted and chopped, 5 large minced garlic cloves, 1/4 cup olive oil, 2 tablespoons fresh lemon juice, 1 tablespoon balsamic vinegar, 2 teaspoons sea salt (taste first!), freshly ground black pepper (to taste), and mix well. Toast 1/4 cup pine nuts in a dry pan on medium-low heat, shaking often this should take less than 5 minutes. Place the tomato mixture in a serving dish, and top with the pine nuts and 1/2 cup chopped fresh basil.

Day 4:

Breakfast: Oatmeal/porridge with fruits

Noon Meal: Winter Lentil Soup

Evening Meal: Stuffed Green Peppers

Stuffed Green Peppers

Ingredients:

- Cooked Brown Rice
- Small Tomatoes
- Frozen Corn
- Sweet Onion
- Ripe Olives
- Canned Black Beans
- Canned Red Beans
- Fresh Basil Leaves
- Garlic Cloves
- Salt
- Pepper
- Vegan Cheese
- Spaghetti Sauce

Instructions:

Combine 2 cups cooked brown rice, 3 small tomatoes, chopped, 1 cup frozen corn, thawed, 1 small sweet onion, chopped, 1 can (4-1/4 ounces) chopped ripe olives, 1/3 cup canned black beans, rinsed and drained, 1/3 cup canned red beans, rinsed and drained, 4 fresh basil leaves, thinly sliced, 3 garlic cloves, minced, 1 teaspoon salt, and 1/2 teaspoon pepper. Add ¾ cup vegan cheese, if desired.

Cut the tops off of 6 large sweet peppers, and remove the seeds, being careful not to break the pepper. Fill each pepper with the rice mixture, and place in a crock pot Cover the bottom of the pot and the peppers with 3/4 cup spaghetti sauce and 1/2 cup water. Cook for 3 ½ to 4 hours on low.

Day 5:

Breakfast: Blueberry/Banana Smoothie- a bit of orange adds zest!

Noon Meal: Sloppy Joe's- with red or brown lentils instead of meat

Evening Meal: Slow-Cooker Jambalaya

Chapter 9: Week Eight

Day 1:

Breakfast: Cereal with ginger, apple, and agave

Noon Meal: Black Bean Quesadillas

Evening Meal: Italian-Inspired Soup

Italian-Inspired Soup

Ingredients:

- Olive Oil
- White Onion
- Carrots
- Celery
- Cloves Garlic
- Vegetable Stock
- Fire-Roasted Tomatoes
- Wheat Pasta
- Dried Thyme
- Dried Oregano
- Rosemary
- Spinach

Instructions:

In a stockpot, heat 2 tablespoons olive oil, and sauté one small white onion until tender. Add 1-cup carrots, cut into rounds, 1-cup celery cut into similar sized pieces, and 3 cloves garlic. Sauté for an additional 3 minutes.

Add 6 cups vegetable stock, a 14 ounce can fire-roasted tomatoes, 8 ounces whole-wheat pasta (orzo is a good choice), 1/2 teaspoon dried thyme, ¼ teaspoon dried oregano and 1/4 teaspoon rosemary, and stir to combine well. After about 10 minutes, add 4 cups spinach. Cook until the spinach is wilted, and test pasta to insure it is done.

Day 2:

Breakfast: Green Smoothie

Green Smoothie

Blend 1-cup berries, 1 handful of greens, a small banana, and orange juice until smooth- adding either water or juice to thin if needed.

Noon Meal: Broccoli and white bean soup- creamy or chunky!

Evening Meal: Vegan pizza

Day 3:

Breakfast: Walnut and spice stuffed apples (make extra to freeze)

Noon Meal: Peanut noodles

Evening Meal: Red Pepper And Pinto Frittata

Red Pepper And Pinto Frittata
Ingredients:

- Pinto Beans
- Red Pepper
- Sweet Onion
- Carrot
- Garlic
- Broccoli
- Plum Tomato
- Chickpea Flour
- Vegetable Stock
- Dried Basil
- Black Salt
- Nutritional Yeast

Instructions:

Pre-cook 1 cup Pinto Beans, drained and rinsed, 1-cup red pepper, chopped, 1 cup sweet onion, chopped, 1/2 cup carrot, grated, 2 tbsp. garlic, minced, 1/2 cup broccoli, divided into mini florets, and 1 plum tomato, diced. These can be left overs. Heat the oven to 400 degrees, and oil a cake pan.

In a small bowl, mix 1-cup chickpea flour with 1-cup water until it is a smooth paste. Bring 1 ½ cups vegetable stock, 1 tablespoon dried basil, ½ teaspoon black salt, and 3 tablespoons nutritional yeast to a boil. Add the chickpea flour mixture, and reduce the heat. Stir constantly until the batter thickens, and cook for another 3 minutes afterwards.

Add the bean and red pepper mixture, folding it in gently. Pour into the oil pan, and bake for 25-30 minutes. Let cool before removing from pan.

Day 4:

Breakfast: Breakfast parfait

Noon Meal: Twice-baked potato boats

Evening Meal: Cucumbers, avocados, and onions in a slightly spicy Asian dressing

Day 5:

Breakfast: Cherry Dumplings

Cherry Dumplings

Ingredients:

- Cherries
- Flour
- Baking Powder
- Sugar
- Vegan Margarine
- Plant Milk

Instructions:

In a deep pan, bring to a gentle boil 2 cups cherries, and 1 cup water, adjusting the sweetness for your taste- they should be just slightly sour to balance the dumpling.

Stir together 2 cups flour, 2 teaspoons baking powder, ½ teaspoon sugar, 2 tablespoons vegan margarine, and ¾ cup plant milk. Scoop out with a teaspoon, and gently drop the dumplings into the pot one at a time, making sure that they are completely covered. Steam with the lid on loosely for 10-15 minutes. Break open the largest of the dumplings, and make sure they are fluffy all the way through. Serve hot, or remove the cherries and store the dumpling separately for later enjoyment. **Noon Meal:** Quinoa with edamame and corn **Evening Meal:** Seven-vegetable couscous

Chapter 10: Week Nine

Day 1:

Breakfast: Tofu Breakfast Scramble

Tofu Breakfast Scramble

Cook 4 ounces of drained tofu and 2 spring onions (or one leek) in a pan with a bit of oil for one minute; add 2 teaspoons tamari, 2 tablespoons savory yeast flakes, ½ teaspoon turmeric, and 2 to 3 tablespoons water and cook for another minute. Serve with toast, has browns, or English muffin,

Noon Meal: Vegetable stew

Evening Meal: Vegan Alfredo With Peas And Kale

Vegan Alfredo With Peas And Kale

Ingredients:

- Minced Garlic Cloves
- Arrowroot Powder
- Plant Milk
- Salt And Pepper
- Nutritional Yeast
- Garlic Powder
- Vegan Parmesan

Instructions:

Sauté 4 minced garlic cloves in oil until tender. Add 4 tablespoons arrowroot powder, and whisk until smooth. Add ¼ cup at a time 1 ¾ cup plant milk, whisking well to avoid lumps. Cook for 2 minutes.

Transfer to a blender, and salt and pepper to taste. Add 4 tablespoons nutritional yeast, and ½ teaspoon garlic powder. Blend on high until creamy. Up to ¼ cup of vegan Parmesan may be added, as well.

Return to pan, and cook on medium heat until it bubbles, then turn the heat to low and continue to cook until it thickens. You may need to add an additional ¼ cup of plant milk, or remove ½ cup of the sauce, and add 1-teaspoon arrowroot whisked well, to thicken more.

Serve over pasta, and top with fresh vegetables.

Day 2:

Breakfast: Jelly Muffin

Noon Meal: Mushroom Pho

Evening Meal: Asparagus and Carrot Indian Stir Fry

Day 3:

Breakfast: Muffin Square

Noon Meal: BLT- sprouts, avocado, fresh basil, tomatoes, and vegan bacon

Evening Meal: Chard, chickpea, and rice casserole

Day 4:

Breakfast: Lemon Scones

Lemon Scones
Ingredients:

- All-Purpose Flour
- Sugar
- Baking Powder
- Baking Soda
- Salt
- Lemon Zest
- Cold Coconut Oil
- Almond Milk
- Lemon Juice
- Apple Cider Vinegar
- Vanilla Extract

Instructions:

Mix together in a large bowl 3 1/4 cup all-purpose flour, 1/2-cup sugar, 1 T baking powder, 1/2 t baking soda, 1 t salt and 2 T lemon zest. Using a pastry cutter or a fork cut in 8 T cold coconut oil until the mixture is evenly crumbly.

In a small bowl, mix 1 1/2 cups almond milk, 1/3 cup lemon juice, and 1 T apple cider vinegar. Let sit for 2 minutes or until the milk begins to curdle. Add 1 t vanilla extract, and pour the liquids into the dry ingredients and mix well. Dough will be sticky, so knead it a few times, and pat into a circle about 2 inches thick on a parchment paper-covered cookie sheet. Brush with almond milk and sprinkle with sugar. Bake in a 400-degree oven for 20 to 25 minutes or until golden brown.

Noon Meal: Chick-less noodle soup

Evening Meal: Vegan Pizza

Day 5:

Breakfast: Strawberry pancakes

Strawberry Pancakes

Ingredients:

- Flour
- Rolled Oats
- Baking Powder
- Salt
- Pure Vanilla Extract
- Sugar
- Plant Milk
- Unrefined Coconut Oil
- Chopped Strawberries
- Fruit Butter

Instructions:

Combine 1/3-cup flour, 2 tbsp. rolled oats, 2/3 tsp. baking powder, and 1/8 tsp. salt. Add 1/2 tsp. pure vanilla extract, 1 tbsp. sugar, 1/3-cup plant milk, and 1 tbsp. unrefined coconut oil. Fold in ½ cup chopped strawberries.

Cook in an oiled pan, turning once. These will cook fairly quickly. Make a fruit compote, or add fruit butter to the top.

Noon Meal: Miso vegetable soup

Evening Meal: Soba noodles with green curry

Transitioning Vegan

BOOK 4

Introduction

Vegetarianism is nothing new. In fact, it has been around since, at least, 580 BC and was even a popular lifestyle choice for Pythagoras, who was an Ionian Greek philosopher and mathematician. Pythagoras was one of the first to admit that animals deserved to be treated well and people should try to abstain from consuming meat. These ideas of Pythagoras were not new, however, and in fact were the same traditions found in some earlier civilizations, like the ancient Egyptians.

Vegetarianism isn't just about animal cruelty, though that is a big reason for many people. It also provides a slew of health benefits that a meat filled diet just cannot give you. Vegetarian diets are actually really low in fat yet high in vegetables and fruits.

Maintaining a vegetarian diet also reduces the chance of suffering from food poison, which occurs millions of times a year due to spoiled meat. Studies have also shown that a meatless diet can help you shed those unwanted pounds. This has to do with several reasons, including replacing meat with more nutritious foods, such as whole grains, fresh fruits, fresh vegetables and beans.

Research has also shown that vegetarians are less likely to experience diseases, such as obesity, coronary heart disease, type two diabetes, high blood pressure and cancers related to diet.

In fact, living a vegan or vegetarian lifestyle can lower the amount of saturated fats while increasing the amount of healthy carbohydrates, fiber, potassium and magnesium you intake.

But what does this mean?

Well, reducing your intake of saturated fats will greatly improve your health, which is especially important if you deal with cardiovascular complications. Increasing healthy carbohydrates, which are naturally found in vegetables, will help prevent muscle mass burn, which essentially means you can maintain a healthy vegan/vegetarian lifestyle while still gaining muscle. And I'm sure you know that a diet high in fiber promotes healthier digestive tract. As for an increase in potassium and magnesium, well, these two vital minerals are essential for a healthy mind and body. Potassium helps to ensure the acidity and water in your body is properly balanced and it helps the kidneys get rid of harmful toxins. Studies have also shown that diets with an abundance of potassium can reduce the risk of cardiovascular dieses and cancer. Magnesium is an often overlook mineral/vitamin that is vital to the proper absorption of calcium. Dark greens, seeds and nuts are a few foods that are naturally high in magnesium.

Despite all the benefits that a vegan/vegetarian lifestyle has, trying to live in a meat eater's world can be more than a little difficult. Not only do you have to regularly explain to close minded people why you are a vegetarian (fielding questions and snide remarks left and right), but you also have to contend with the vegetarian diet, which can be more than a little daunting, especially for those new to this massive lifestyle change. After all, you are going against the traditional diet that is considered the traditional or normal way to live. Just turn on your television and after an hour you will have been bombarded with ads designed to entice the wild meat eating beast that lurks in all of use. But just because the initial transitioning is hard doesn't mean you cannot be successful.

That is where this vegetarian cookbook comes in handy. Not only does it provide the reader with 31 of the best recipes, it also gives you step-by-step instructions that even the most novice chef can follow.

A lot of people overlook the vegetarian lifestyle because they think it's too hard or takes too much time, which, let's face it, most people just don't have in their busy, fast-paced life. And while it is true that maintaining a vegetarian lifestyle can be a bit difficult at first, the benefits that you receive from living it is so worth it that you will wonder why you didn't come over to the plant-side sooner.

This vegetarian cookbook will help you in your journey into the wonderful world of vegetarianism. Inside this book, you will find recipes for every meal of the day, including breakfast, lunch and dinner. You will also find delicious smoothie, shake, juice and dessert recipes that won't break your vegetarian lifestyle.

So what are you waiting for? Start reading Chapter 1 now!

Chapter 1: Vegetarian Breakfast Recipes

The following breakfast recipes are designed to start your day off right while still maintaining your vegetarian lifestyle. Remember, breakfast is the most important meal of the day and you shouldn't skip it if at all possible.

Whole Wheat Pancakes

Serves: 4 to 5

Ingredients:

- 1 cup flour, whole wheat
- 1/3 cup wheat germ
- 2/3 cup flour, all-purpose
- 2 tablespoons brown sugar
- 1 teaspoon table salt
- ½ teaspoon baking soda
- 1 ½ teaspoon baking powder
- 2 large eggs, beaten
- 5 1/3 tablespoons butter, unsalted
- 2 ½ cups buttermilk

Directions:

Step 1: Combine the both flours, wheat germ, sugar, baking powder, baking soda and salt together in a mixing bowl.

Cut in the butter and continue to mix until it achieves a consistency similar to sand.

Step 2: Make a hole in the middle of the mixture. Pour the beaten eggs and buttermilk into the hole and mix until well combined.

Step 3: Use the batter to make the whole wheat pancakes as you normally would. Top with your favorite toppings, such as organic maple syrup or fruit.

Breakfast Casserole featuring Sweet Potatoes

Serves: 12

Ingredients:

- 1 8-ounce package vegetarian sausage, cooked
- ¼ cup butter, melted
- ½ cup water
- 4 cups sweet potatoes, shredded
- ½ cup onions, chopped finely
- 1 ½ 8-ounce package mozzarella/cheddar cheese blend
- 8 eggs, large
- 1 cup spinach, sliced
- 1 16-ounce container cottage cheese, small curd

Directions:

Step 1: Preheat the oven to 350-degrees and lightly grease a baking dish. Crumble the cooked vegetarian sausage into a bowl.

Step 2: Mix the melted butter and the shredded sweet potatoes together before spreading it into the baking dish from Step 1.

Step 3: Combine the cheese blend, eggs, sausage, onions and spinach together. Spread this mixture evenly over the butter/potato mixture.

Step 4: Place the baking dish in the oven and cook for about 20 minutes. Remove from the oven and let cool for a few minutes before serving.

Apple Wraps

Serves: 2

Ingredients:

- 2 whole wheat tortillas
- ¼ cup organic apple butter
- 2 cups green apples, cored/peeled/diced
- 1 cup rolled oats
- 1 teaspoon vanilla extract
- 1 tablespoon butter
- 1 ½ cup almond milk
- 1 teaspoon cinnamon
- 1/8 teaspoon salt
- ¼ cup organic raisins
- ¼ cup organic honey

Directions:

Step 1: Mix the honey, salt, cinnamon and raisins together. Add the apples and toss until coated.

Step 2: Melt the butter in a large saucepan. Add the coated apple and cook over medium heat for about 8 to 10 minutes. Make sure to stir occasionally. You want the apples to be tender.

Step 3: Stir in the milk and oatmeal before turning the heat down a bit and allowing to mixture to cook for about 5 minutes.

Step 4: Remove the saucepan from heat and stir in the vanilla. Evenly spread some organic apple butter on the tortillas before spooning the cooked mixture on top of the apple butter.

Step 5: Wrap the tortillas and serve warm.

Breakfast Green Smoothie

Serves: 1

Ingredients:

- 2 kale leaves
- 2 carrots
- 2 celery sticks
- 1 pear, remove core and slice into small pieces
- 1 knob ginger, small
- 2 cups baby spinach
- 1 tablespoons chia seeds
- 6 ice cubes

Directions:

Step 1: Place all ingredients into a blender and blend until smooth, which should be about 30 to 60 seconds.

Step 2: Pour the smoothie into a glass and enjoy.

Oatmeal and Blueberry Waffles

Serves: 3

Ingredients:

- 1 cup flour, whole wheat
- ½ teaspoon salt
- 1 tablespoon baking powder
- ¼ teaspoon allspice
- 1 cup oats, quick cooking
- 1/3 cup organic applesauce, unsweetened
- 1 ½ cups almond milk, unsweetened
- 2 tablespoons canola oil
- 3 tablespoons real maple syrup
- 1 teaspoon vanilla extract
- 1 ½ cup blueberries, frozen

Directions:

Step 1: Sift the baking powder, flour, allspice and salt together in a mixing bowl. Stir in the oats. Create a small well in the middle of the mixture and add the milk, applesauce, vanilla, oil and maple syrup into the whole. Mix until all ingredients are well combined.

Step 2: Allow the mixture to sit undisturbed for about 5 minutes. Gently fold the frozen blueberries into the mixture.

Step 3: Pour about ½ cup of the mixture into a heated waffle iron and cook until the waffle is done. Repeat with the remaining batter. Serve the waffles with your favorite toppings.

Chapter 2: Vegetarian Lunch Recipes

While the following vegetarian recipes are designed for lunchtime, you can make them at any time of the day.

Salsa and Black Bean Soup

Serves: 4

Ingredients:

- 2 cans black beans, drained and rinsed
- 1 cup salsa, chunky
- 1 ½ cup organic vegetable broth
- 1 teaspoon cumin
- 2 ½ tablespoons green onions, sliced

Directions:

Step 1: Pour the beans, vegetable broth, cumin and salsa into a blender and blend until the mixture is almost smooth.

Step 2: Pour the mixture into a large saucepan and place on the stove over medium heat. Heat until the mixture is completely heated.

Step 3: Divide the soup between 4 soup bowls and top with some sliced green onions.

Carrot and Lentil Soup

Serves: 2

Ingredients:

- 3 ounces red lentils
- 1 cube vegetable stock, crumbled
- 3 garlic cloves, sliced
- 2 carrots, cleaned and diced
- 2 teaspoons olive oil
- 1 onion, sliced finely
- 2 tablespoons parsley, chopped

Directions:

Step 1: Heat the oil in a saucepan. While the oil is heating, bring 1 liter of water to a boil.

Step 2: Add the chopped onions into the heated oil and fry for a few minutes. Add in the garlic and carrots.

Step 3: Carefully pour the boiling water into the saucepan with the onions, garlic and carrots. Stir in the vegetable stock cube and the lentils. Let cook for about 15 minutes.

Step 4: Remove the saucepan from heat and stir in the parsley. Spoon the soup into the bowls and serve while warm.

Tofu Lunch Scramble

Serves: 4

Ingredients:

- 1 14-ounce package tofu, rinsed
- 3 teaspoons canola oil, divided in half
- 1 teaspoon cumin
- 1 ½ teaspoons chili powder
- ½ teaspoon salt, divide in half
- ¾ cup corn
- 1 zucchini, diced
- 4 scallions, diced
- ½ cup salsa
- ½ cup shredded cheese
- ¼ cup cilantro, chopped

Directions:

Step 1: Place 1 ½ teaspoon of the oil into a large skillet. Warm the oil over medium heat. Stir in the tofu, cumin, chili powder and ¼ teaspoon of salt. Cook for about 6 minutes or until the tofu starts to turn a brownish color. When this occurs, transfer the mixture to a bowl.

Step 2: Mix in the remaining ingredients until everything is well combined. Divide the scramble between 4 dishes and serve immediately.

Fried Tofu and Mushrooms Served in Lettuce Cups

Serves: 6

Ingredients:

- 10 ¾ ounce shitake mushrooms, dried and chopped
- 1 tablespoon lime juice
- 2 tablespoons hoisin sauce
- 2 tablespoons roasted peanut oil
- 3 minced garlic cloves
- 1 Thai chili, seeds removed and diced
- 1 tablespoon minced ginger root
- 12 ounces tofu, drained and diced
- 12 lettuce leaves

Directions:

Step 1: Place a cup of hot water in a bowl and add the dried mushrooms. Let the mushrooms soak for about 10 minutes. Strain the liquid from the mushrooms and mix them the hoisin sauce.

Step 2: Coat a saucepan with the peanut oil and heat on the stove over medium heat. Place the mushrooms, ginger, chili and garlic into the heated pan and cook for a few minutes.

Step 3: Place the tofu into the pan and cook for several minutes. You want the tofu to have a light brown color.

Step 4: Spoon the cooked tofu mixture into the 12 lettuce leaves. Roll the leaves up and serve immediately.

Lunch Beans in a Crockpot

Serves: 4

Ingredients:

- 1 onion, diced
- 1 pound cannellini beans, dried
- 4 garlic cloves, minced
- 1 bay leaf
- 1 teaspoon thyme, dried
- ½ teaspoon salt, table or kosher
- 5 cups boiling water

Directions:

Step 1: Place the beans in a large pot filled with cold water. The beans should be completely covered by the water.

Let the beans soak for at least 6 hours but preferably overnight.

Step 2: Drain the beans from the water and place them inside crockpot. Stir in the diced onions, minced garlic cloves, bay leaf and thyme. Pour the boiling water overtop the ingredients. Place the cover on the crockpot and cook for 3 ½ hours.

Step 3: Add the salt and stir before placing the lid back n the crockpot and cooking and additional 15 minutes.

Tomato Basil Crockpot Soup

Serves: 4

Ingredients:

- 10 basil leaves, fresh
- 12 tomatoes, diced
- 6 ounce can tomato paste
- 1 tablespoon vegan butter
- ¼ teaspoon ground black pepper
- 1 tablespoon Italian seasoning
- 2 cups soy milk
- 2 tablespoons flour, whole wheat

Directions:

Step 1: Place the basil leaves, diced tomatoes, tomato paste and ground pepper into the crockpot.

Step 2: In a small bowl, whisk together the whole wheat flour and soy milk. Pour the mixture into the crockpot.

Step 3: Place the lid on the crockpot and cook on low for about 6 hours.

Step 4: Transfer the soup into a food processor and pulse for several seconds. You want the soup to have a little chunkiness to it. Place the soup make into the crockpot and keep warm until ready to serve.

Chapter 3: Vegetarian Dinner Recipes

If you find yourself searching for a vegetarian recipe to feed a large amount of people, simple double (or triple) the ingredients of these following dinner recipes, which will please both vegetarians and meat eaters a like.

Stuffed Peppers

Serves: 6

Ingredients:

- 2 cups brown rice, cooked
- 1 cup frozen corn, thawed
- 3 small tomatoes, diced
- 1 sweet onion, diced
- ¾ cup vegan cheese substitute
- 1/3 cup canned black beans, rinsed with water and drained
- 4 ¼ ounce ripe olives, chopped
- 1/3 cup canned red beans, rinsed with water and drained
- 3 garlic cloves, minced
- 4 fresh basil leaves, sliced thinly
- ½ teaspoon black pepper
- 1 teaspoon salt
- ¾ cup spaghetti sauce, meatless
- 6 sweet peppers, large
- ½ cup water

Directions:

Step 1: Mix the brown rice, tomatoes, corn, onion, cheese substitute, olives, beans, basil leaves, garlic cloves, salt and pepper together in a bowl.

Step 2: Cut the top of the sweet peppers off and remove the seeds inside. Stuff the peppers with the mixture from Step 1.

Step 3: Mix the meatless spaghetti sauce and water together. Pour half of this mixture into a crockpot. Place the stuffed peppers into the crockpot and pour the remaining water/sauce mixture on top.

Step 4: Place the lid on the crockpot and cook on low for 4 hours.

Cauliflower Tacos

Serves: 4 to 8

Ingredients:

- 1 cauliflower head
- 2 tablespoons olive oil, divided
- 1 can chickpeas
- 1 teaspoon salt, divided
- ¼ teaspoon cumin
- ¼ teaspoon chili powder
- 1 garlic clove, minced
- 2 cups cilantro, fresh
- 8 tortillas

Directions:

Step 1: Preheat the oven to 425-degrees. Cut the head of cauliflower into florets. Place the florets in a bowl and drizzle with 1 tablespoon olive oil and ½ teaspoon of salt. Spread the covered florets onto a baking sheet and bake for about 15 minutes. You want to brown the florets.

Step 2: While the florets are in the oven, mix the remaining salt, chickpeas, cumin and chili powder together in a bowl. Stir in the remaining olive oil. Spread the mixture onto a clean baking sheet and place in the oven for 15 minutes.

Step 3: Evenly divide the garlic and cilantro between the tortillas. Add ½ cup of the florets mixture and 1 teaspoon of the chickpea mixture to the tortillas. Roll the tortillas up and serve.

Bean Burgers Smokey-Style

Serves: 2

Ingredients:

- ½ cup sunflower seeds, coarsely chopped
- 1/3 cup oats, quick cooking
- ½ green bell pepper, diced
- 1 can pinto beans, drained and rinsed
- ½ cup hemp seeds
- 1 teaspoon chili powder
- 2 teaspoons salt
- 1 teaspoon paprika
- 1 tablespoon olive oil
- Salt and black pepper to taste
- Lettuce, tomatoes, onions and other toppings and/or condiments (optional)
- Hamburger buns, whole grain

Directions:

Step 1: Preheat the oven to 400-degrees. Mix the quick cooking oats with 2/3 cup of boiling water.

Step 2: Mix the hemp seeds, beans, bell pepper, olive oil and seasonings together in a bowl. Place the mixture in a food processor and process for several seconds.

Step 3: Transfer the pulsed mixture into a bowl and stir in the oatmeal and sunflower seeds.

Step 4: Coat the bottom of a baking sheet with olive oil. Scoop the mixture out of the bowl using a measuring cup.

Pat the mixture into a patty shape. Place the patty on the baking sheet.

Step 5: Place the baking sheet in the oven and bake for 15 minutes. Flip the patties and allow to bake for an additional 15 minutes.

Step 6: Serve the vegetarian burgers on whole grain bread with your desired toppings.

Rigatoni and Sautéed Vegetables

Serves: 2 to 4

Ingredients:

- 5 ½ cups rigatoni, cooked and drained according to the package instructions
- 1 eggplant, cut into bite-sized pieces
- 3 tablespoons olive oil
- 1 pint cherry tomatoes, cut in half
- 3 garlic cloves, thinly sliced
- ¼ cup fresh mint, torn into pieces
- Pinch of salt, table or kosher
- Pinch of black pepper

Directions:

Step 1: Place the oil in a skillet and heat over high heat. Add the pieces of eggplant, salt and pepper. Cook for about 10 minutes or until the eggplant develops a brown color. Make sure to stir the cooking eggplant occasionally.

Step 2: Stir in the halved tomatoes and garlic and cook for an additional 4 minutes. Add the cooked and drained rigatoni and the mint. Mix until all is well combined.

Step 3: Divide the meal between the serving bowls and enjoy.

Vegetarian Chili with a dash of Chocolate

Serves: 4

Ingredients:

- 1 ½ ounces chocolate, bittersweet
- 1 teaspoon salt
- 1 tablespoon olive oil
- 2 teaspoons cumin
- 1 garlic clove, minced
- 1 green pepper, diced
- 1 white onion, chopped finely
- 2 tomatoes, diced
- 2 cans kidney beans, drained and rinsed
- 2 cans chickpeas, drained and rinsed
- 5 cups vegetable broth

Directions:

Step 1: Place the oil in a large pot. Set the pot on the stove over high heat. Add the garlic, green pepper and onion.
Cook until the vegetables have begun to soften, which is generally about 5 minutes.

Step 2: Stir in the kidney beans, chickpeas, cumin, salt, tomatoes and vegetable broth. Let the mixture cook and bring it to a boil. Once it begins to boil, turn the heat to low, cover the pot and let the mixture simmer.

Step 3: Allow the mixture to cook for about an hour or until it starts to thicken. Stir in the chocolate and continue to cook until it has completely melted.

Step 4: Divide the vegetarian chili between the serving bowls and enjoy.

Vegetarian Sloppy Joes

Serves: 4

Ingredients:

- ½ cup quinoa
- 1 yellow onion, diced
- 1 tablespoon olive oil
- 1 ½ cup pinto beans, drained and rinsed
- ½ green pepper, diced
- 1 can tomato sauce
- 1 tablespoon soy sauce
- 1 tomato, diced
- 2 teaspoons chili powder
- ¼ teaspoon oregano, dried
- ½ teaspoon paprika
- Rolls, whole grain

Directions:

Step 1: In a small pot, mix 1 cup of water with the quinoa. Bring the mixture to a boil before reducing the heat and covering the pot. Let the mixture simmer for about 15 minutes.

Step 2: Place the olive oil in a skillet. Sauté the diced onion for a few minutes. Stir in the green pepper and continue to sauté until the vegetables are tender.

Step 3: Stir in the remaining ingredients except for the whole grain rolls. Let the ingredients cook for about 5 minutes. Remove the mixture from heat and let sit for an additional 5 minutes.

Step 4: Stir in the mixture from step 1 and let sit for another 5 minutes. Scoop the mixture onto the whole grain rolls and serve with a side of your favorite vegetables or salad.

Pad Thai Noodles

Serves: 3 to 4

Ingredients:

- 1 package rice noodles, cooked according to the directions on the package
- ½ cup peanut butter
- 1 cup coconut milk
- 2 garlic cloves, minced
- 1 tablespoon ginger, fresh
- ¼ cup lime juice
- ½ teaspoon salt, table or kosher
- 1 teaspoon chili sauce
- ½ teaspoon peanut oil
- 1 cup tofu
- 1 red pepper, diced
- 2 cups shitake mushrooms, sliced
- 1 cup snow peas
- 1 cup broccoli florets
- 1 cup baby bok choy, chopped
- ½ cup peanuts, roasted
- Olive oil

Directions:

Step 1: Mix the peanut butter, coconut milk, ginger, salt, garlic, peanut oil, lime juice and chili sauce together. Set to the side for the moment.

Step 2: In a pan, heat the olive oil. Add the tofu and cook until it is brown on all sides. Remove the tofu from the pan and set to the side for the moment.

Step 3: Add 1 teaspoon of olive oil to the pan and sauté the mushrooms, broccoli florets, snow peas and bell pepper for about 10 minutes.

Step 4: Stir in the bok choy and browned tofu. Cook for an additional 2 minutes.

Step 5: Divide the cooked noodles between the serving dishes. Add the browned tofu and bok choy. Drizzle the mixture from Step 1 over the top and garnish with roasted peanuts.

Vegetarian Pizza

Serves: Makes 2 9x18-inches pizzas

Ingredients:

- 2 teaspoons red peppers, diced
- 2 eggplants, diced
- ½ cup olive oil, extra virgin
- 2 pounds frozen pizza dough
- 3 cups shredded mozzarella vegan substitute
- 1 ½ cups tomato sauce
- Fresh basil
- Pinch salt, table or kosher
- Pinch black pepper
- Sweet potatoes

Directions:

Step 1: Turn the grill on and let heat at a medium to high temperature.

Step 2: Toss all the vegetables with ¼ cup of the olive oil. Season with salt and pepper.

Step 3: Grill the coated vegetables in batches until they are soft but still have a bit of crunch to them. Place the grilled vegetables to the side.

Step 4: Roll the pizza dough out to make 2 9x18-inch pizzas that are about 1/8-inch thick.

Step 5: Brush one side of the pizza with 1 tablespoon of olive oil. Do the same for the second pizza. Season the pizza with salt and pepper. Place the pizzas, oil-side down, onto the grill. Grill for about 9 minutes.

Step 6: Repeat Step 5 with the opposite side of the pizzas.

Step 7: Evenly spread the pizza sauce over one side of each pizza. Top with the vegan cheese substitute and grilled vegetables. Close the lid of the grill and let the cheese substitute melt. Garnish with fresh basil before cutting the pizzas into slices.

Chapter 4: Vegetarian Smoothie, Shakes and Juice Recipes

The following smoothie, shakes and juice recipes can be used as a meal substitute or for when you're craving something but don't want a big meal. In fact, the following recipes work great as an on-the-go breakfast meal when you just don't have the time to prepare and sit down to eat a traditional breakfast meal.

Banana and Ginger Smoothie

Serves: 1

Ingredients:

- 1 ripe banana, sliced
- 1 tablespoon honey
- 1 cup vanilla vegan yogurt
- ½ teaspoon grated ginger

Directions:

Step 1: Place all 4 ingredients into a blender and blend until the mixture is smooth. Pour the smoothie into a tall glass and enjoy.

Purple Power Smoothie

Serves: 1

Ingredients:

- ½ cup blueberries
- 1 ¼ cup milk, soy
- ½ banana
- 1 teaspoon vanilla extract
- 2 teaspoons sugar

Directions:

Step 1: Place all the ingredients into a blender and blend until smooth. Pour the smoothie into a glass and enjoy.

Chocolate and Cherry Shake

Serves: 1

Ingredients:

- 12 ounces soy milk
- 2 scoops protein powder, chocolate flavor
- 2 cups cherries, pitted
- 1 tablespoon walnuts
- 1 cup baby spinach
- 1 tablespoon dark cocoa powder
- 1 tablespoon ground flax

Directions:

Step 1: Add all ingredients into a blender and blend until smooth. Transfer the shake into a glass and enjoy.

Green Detox Smoothie

Serves: 1

Ingredients:

- 1 kiwi, peeled
- ½ cup pineapple, chopped
- 1 cup coconut water
- Handful baby spinach
- ½ avocado, peeled and chopped
- 1 teaspoon coconut oil

Directions:

Step 1: Add all ingredients into a blender and blend until smooth. Transfer the detox smoothie into a glass and enjoy.

Berry Strawberry Smoothie

Serves: 1

Ingredients:

- 2 cups strawberries, stems removed
- 2 basil springs
- 1 handful mint
- 1 ripe banana
- ½ cup apple juice
- 1 teaspoon honey

Directions:

Step 1: Add all ingredients into a blender and blend until smooth. Transfer the shake into a glass and enjoy.

Pumpkin Pie Smoothie

Serves: 1

Ingredients:

- 1 cup almond milk
- 1 cup pumpkin puree
- 1 teaspoon agave nectar
- 1 red apple, cored
- 2 teaspoons cinnamon
- Handful cranberries, dried

Directions:

Step 1: Add all ingredients into a blender and blend until smooth. Transfer the shake into a glass and enjoy.

Antioxidant Boost Smoothie

Serves: 1

Ingredients:

- ½ cup acia berry puree
- ½ cup pomegranate arils
- 1 ripe banana
- ½ cup blueberries
- 8 ounces almond milk

Directions:

Step 1: Add all ingredients into a blender and blend until smooth. Transfer the shake into a glass and enjoy.

Golden Delicious Juice

Serves: 1

Ingredients:

- 4 stalks celery
- 2 carrots
- ½ cucumber
- 1 pear
- ½ cup beetroot
- Sprinkle ginger, diced

Directions:

Step 1: Place all ingredients into a blender. Blend for several seconds or until the ingredients are smooth.

Step 2: Pour the juice into a glass and enjoy immediately.

Chapter 5: Vegetarian Dessert Recipes

Yes, even vegetarians can make and enjoy delicious desserts while still maintaining their vegetarian lifestyle. And these yummy dessert recipes prove just that!

Chocolate and Banana Mousse

Serves: 4

Ingredients:

- 1 cup semi-sweet chocolate chips
- 2 bananas, ripe
- 10 ounce tofu, silken soft
- 3 tablespoons brown sugar
- 1 teaspoon vanilla extract
- 1 teaspoon raspberry vinegar
- ¼ teaspoon salt

Directions:

Step 1: In a microwave safe bowl, melt the chocolate chips.

Step 2: Place half the banana and the tofu into a blender and blend until the two ingredients are smooth. Add the other half of the banana and blend until smooth.

Step 3: Add in the brown sugar, raspberry vinegar, salt and vanilla extract and blend until smooth. Transfer the melted chocolate chips into the blender and blender once more.

Step 4: Scoop the mixture out of the blender and into an air tight container. Place the container in the fridge and chill for at least 3 hours before consuming.

Simple Fruit Cocktail Cake

Serves: 6

Ingredients:

- 9 ounce package yellow cake mix
- 1 can fruit cocktail packed in light syrup

Directions:

Step 1: Preheat the oven to 350-degrees. Light grease the inside of a baking pan that measures 9x9-inches.

Step 2: Drain the fruit cocktail, pouring the syrup into a mixing bowl. Add the cake mix and combined until well mixed.

Step 3: Gently mix in the fruit cocktail. Spread the mixture into the prepared baking pan. Place the pan in the oven and bake for about 45 minutes.

Biscotti al Pistachio

Serves: 2 dozen cookies

Ingredients:

- 500 grams raw pistachios
- 1 teaspoon vanilla extract
- 200 grams white sugar
- 1 ½ teaspoon lemon zest
- 1 tablespoon honey
- Powdered sugar

Directions:

Step 1: Place the pistachios into a food processor and pulse until they are finely chopped.

Step 2: Transfer the chopped pistachios into a mixing bowl. Stir in the white sugar, lemon zest, vanilla extract and honey. This is the dough.

Step 3: Roll the dough into small balls and cover them with powdered sugar. Place the dough onto a parchment paper-lined cookie sheet.

Step 4: Place the cookie sheets into a oven preheated at 350-degrees. Bake for 16 to 18 minutes.

Pumpkin and Pear Dessert Bread

Serves: 1 loaf

Ingredients:

- 1 cup all-purpose flour
- 1 ¼ cup white sugar
- 1 cup whole wheat flour
- 2 teaspoon cinnamon
- 2 teaspoon baking powder
- 1 teaspoon baking soda
- ¼ teaspoon table or kosher salt
- ½ cup milk, almond, coconut or soy
- ¾ cup pumpkin puree
- ½ cup vegetable oil
- 1 15-ounce can pears, drained and diced
- 1 teaspoon real vanilla extract

Directions:

Step 1: Preheat the oven to 350-degrees. Spray a 9-inch loaf pan with cooking spray. Set the pan to the side for the moment.

Step 2: Mix the sugar, baking powder, baking soda, cinnamon, salt and flour together. Place to the side for the moment.

Step 3: In a second mixing bowl, combined the vanilla, milk, oil and pumpkin puree. Add in the flour mixture from step 2. Fold in the pears.

Step 4: Pour the batter into the prepared pan from Step 1. Place the loaf pan in the preheated oven and bake for 55 minutes or until a toothpick inserted into the center of the bread comes out clean.

Step 5: Let the bread cool for several minutes before cutting and serving.

CPSIA information can be obtained
at www.ICGtesting.com
Printed in the USA
BVHW070858150321
602550BV00010B/1108